Taming the Beast

Disclaimer

The information written in this book is designed to provide helpful information on fibromyalgia and the subjects discussed. This book is not meant to be used to diagnose or treat any medical condition, or to replace the advice of your physician(s). The authors of this book do not claim to have found a cure for fibromyalgia or any other specific condition.

The reader should regularly consult a physician in matters relating to his or her health, particularly with respect to any symptoms that may require diagnosis or medical attention. For diagnosis or treatment of any medical problem, consult your own physician(s).

The publisher and authors are not responsible or liable for any damages or negative consequences from any treatment, action, application, or preparation to any person reading or following the information in this book. References are provided for informational purposes only and do not constitute endorsement of any websites or other sources. Readers should be aware that the websites listed in this book may change.

This book is dedicated to those in severe chronic daily pain whose lives are not as good as they could be or should be. Those who, despite having been told that there is no hope of recovery, still had enough curiosity, desire for knowledge, and perhaps hope to buy this book. Thank you for not giving up.

I sincerely hope that your journey to health has a happy ending.

Taming the Beast

A GUIDE TO CONQUERING FIBROMYALGIA

DR. KATINKA VAN DER MERWE

CONTENTS

"You treat a disease, you win, you loose. You treat a person, I guarantee you, you'll win, no matter what the outcome."

—Patch Adams

FOREWORD

Let me first take a second to congratulate you for picking up yet another book about your condition. If your life were different, I am sure you would be doing something more fun right now. For whatever reason, you or your loved one was put on a life path that included fibromyalgia. Yet paths may fork, and every journey begins with a single step, as the old Chinese proverb says. If you are reading this, it is for a reason. I trust that it will be worth your while.

Whether you or a family member suffers from fibromyalgia, I sincerely hope that this book will give you some of the answers you have long been searching for about your own condition or perhaps provide you with tools to help better understand the pain and symptoms of someone you care about. As a friend or family member of someone with fibromyalgia, there is no greater gift you can give them than the gift of compassion and caring. Knowledge leads to sympathy and better understanding, and being able to support them better.

The goal of this book is multi-purposed. As a person who suffers from fibromyalgia, you have probably found that much in your life is no longer under your control. You have probably been to a lot of doctors over time, many of whom may not have understood your condition. In addition, fatigue and pain may have robbed you of many of the pleasurable things you once enjoyed.

Overall, it is my hope for you to gain a sense of control over this condition. I want you to walk away from this book empowered. In order to do this, we will lead you through what we believe causes fibromyalgia, its history and its inner workings. In addition, we will provide you with practical steps that will allow you to beat this beast down. We hope to provide you with brand-new, practical information.

Before we delve in, I first want to discuss some of the unique characteristics surrounding fibromyalgia. These make it one of the most difficult, challenging, and complicated conditions to work with and to suffer from.

- Lots of people don't believe in fibromyalgia or don't believe that it's a "real" condition. Unfortunately, those people may include your doctor. Isn't it unfair? After all, it's not like you are asking anyone to believe in alien abductions or in your religion. You just want people to understand that what you are suffering from is as much of a reality as food poisoning is. It *is* real, and it's called suffering every day.

- In general, doctors are very confused about fibromyalgia. It is simply managed as a group of symptoms to be numbed and suppressed. Often, you may be given useless or vague advice. "Take this antidepressant and just try and exercise. Maybe just try to take a walk. Swimming is great exercise. The more you stay active, the better." Does this sound familiar? (Oh, wow. Thanks, doc. What useful information! Next time you have the flu, let's go walk a mile, shall we?) Be patient with your doctor(s) if you can. Even though this type of advice is annoying, it helps to remember that most doctors mean well. Truly, they do—even though it does not make their advice any more helpful or less insulting at times, unfortunately.

- Doctors "treat" fibromyalgia by throwing drugs at it. These drugs (at best) cover up symptoms. In the case of fibromyalgia, it's usually far from the perfect solution, although it may provide some relief. I have yet to meet any patient who told me that him or her, or someone they knew, was "cured" by any drug. Furthermore, every drug has side effects. That being said, I understand that drugs may feel like your only saving grace right now, and that for some of you they are lifesavers. They may make the difference between you getting out of bed in the morning and (kind of) living a halfway normal life, and not.

- People who suffer from fibromyalgia often feel all alone and even ashamed. They feel that some people may think that they just want sympathy, or that it's all in their heads. They may feel that fibromyalgia is still considered the disease of atten- tion-mongers and hypochondriacs. Hardly anyone is organiz- ing marathons or other fundraisers for fibromyalgia. No one is selling purple tubes of lipstick so that a percentage of that sale can be donated to fibromyalgia research. When was the last time you saw someone proudly wearing that little purple ribbon? It's not as popular or sympathy-provoking a cause as breast cancer, and yet it can ruin your life just as surely and methodically. Unfortunately, though, there is still a perceived stigma surrounding fibromyalgia. Let's be honest: as far as dis- eases and conditions go, fibromyalgia is not a trendy or popu- lar one.

- Often, your family and friends don't understand. It doesn't matter how much they love you or how supportive they are. At the end of the day, living with fibromyalgia is like living on an island all alone. It's not a fun island, either. There is no turquoise water, coconuts, white sand, or yummy drinks with tiny umbrellas. Instead, it's a hell on earth. No one can climb inside your body and feel the pain you suffer from every day or understand how life-robbing it is.

- Most of the medical profession (and therefore the public) is of the opinion that it is an incurable condition and a life sentence of pain. Often, when people *do* get better, against all odds, they may be ostracized by the online fibromyalgia community or local support groups as not having had "real" fibromyalgia in the first place, since recovery is clearly not supposed to be possible.

- Fibromyalgia patients themselves often do not fully understand all the symptoms that may be associated with their condition. Knee replacements, anyone? Shoulder problems? Can't stand the noise of a baby crying? Peeing in your pants (*gasp*) at work? Yes. It may all be related.

It isn't fair. I know. If you suffered from, let's say, migraines, you wouldn't have to go around educating the world about your condition and assuring them that yes, migraines *are* real. Why should you have to? Sadly, right now (as a friend of mine is fond of saying), it is what it is, and if you are forced to educate everyone, you may as well get really good at it.

I believe the first step toward educating your family and friends about fibromyalgia is to understand it yourself. It is my hope that this book will assist you in that process.

MY STORY

> *Most men lead lives of quiet desperation and
> go to the grave with the song still in them.*
> —Henry David Thoreau
>
> *Nothing is as important as passion. No matter what
> you want to do with your life, be passionate.*
> —Jon Bon Jovi

I am not sure what your spiritual beliefs are. One of mine, which I hold sacred, is this: that each of us was put upon this earth with a very specific mission and purpose. I believe that we are *meant* to make a difference and to make the world a better place, and that we are meant to live our passion and touch others' lives with it. This is the story of how I found mine.

I was born and raised in Johannesburg, South Africa. I was blessed to have been born to a chiropractic dad and a mother who, once she was exposed to a natural health style, really embraced the philosophy of healthy organic eating and preventative care. Except for emergencies, I was raised with the philosophy that the body is a self-healing, self-regulating organism and can usually heal without medications or shots. The only time we kids would see the doctor was when my brothers needed stitches—which, given that they were typical boys, was quite often.

My family's love of chiropractic is deeply rooted. When my father was seven- years- old, my grandmother was told not to expect him to survive into adulthood, due to very severe allergies. At the time, my grandfather, a very hard working cattle rancher, had been saved from back surgery by a local chiropractor, after his brothers literally carried him out of the hospital into the chiropractor's office. My grandparents wondered if chiropractic care could perhaps help my dad, and they took him along the next time my grandfather had an appointment. Sixty-seven years later, my dad is still very much alive and allergy-free.

Because my dad's life was saved by chiropractic, he felt passionately "called" into that profession. When he was twenty-one, he left South Africa to attend Palmer College of Chiropractic in Davenport, Iowa. He graduated at the age of twenty-four, at which time he went back to South Africa and went on to become extremely successful.

When I was three years old, I climbed onto my dad's big chair behind his desk and announced to my parents that I would be a chiropractor one day. From that point on, I never considered another career. (As it turned out, I became a pretty good oil artist. People would urge me to study art and sell my paintings. I resisted, resolute in my career of choice.) I started chiropractic school in Johannesburg in 1994.

When my family immigrated to the United States in 1994, my dad left behind a thriving practice and many beloved patients. Part of the reason we moved here was because my dad always said that, while he was helping about eight out of every ten patients, he found himself more consumed by the two out of ten whom he *couldn't* help. Eventually, helping those patients with more complicated conditions became an obsession for him, which I in turn inherited. He felt that moving to the United States would afford him with more opportunities to stay on the cutting edge of treatments, techniques, research, and training.

Leaving school, I joined my dad in practice in northwest Arkansas, close to where Walmart is headquartered. It is a lovely, thriving area, and yet I considered it to be only a pit stop while I figured out where in the United States I wanted to settle. After all, I have always lived around big cities. As it turned out, I never left. Later, my younger sister joined us in practice.

From the beginning, practicing as a chiropractor was disappointing to me. I quickly became burned out. Teaching a natural, preventative approach to health (as is the chiropractic school of thought), rather than practicing disease care, is incredibly frustrating. My patients were bombarded by pharmaceutical companies using relentless marketing tools. An age-old model for this is used very successfully: create fear, then offer a solution (for example, create fear of the flu, then offer this season's flu vaccine). In addition, most people had little interest in eating a healthier diet or exercising or investing in preventative health tools such as vitamins and chiropractic.

Another frustrating thing was the type of patients I was treating. While most of them were lovely, I found myself plodding along in mind-numbing symptom mud, consisting of back pain, neck pain, herniated discs, sciatica, and the occasional headache. Fibromyalgia patients were the worst! I noticed that they were much more difficult to treat. Frustratingly, they didn't respond to my care as my other patients did. In addition, these patients were typically taking tons of medications, and overall they just seemed difficult to treat. I dreaded working with them and would often discuss with other doctors whether they thought fibromyalgia was even a real condition or whether it might be psychosomatic. Meanwhile, I lumbered on in practice. My soul longed for more. I needed some purpose. I needed something bigger than myself.

For eight years I practiced like this. I was deeply unhappy and trying to deny it. All around me, I heard chiropractic and spiritual gurus talk about "finding your purpose" and "living passionately." How

I wanted that...my soul cried out for it, but in practice, that was not my reality. I went as far as writing out a mission statement and hanging it above my desk. It described in detail how passionate I was about my work and how I was helping people. The only problem was that I could not lie to myself; deep down, I knew I was a fraud.

You see, chiropractors typically walk a difficult path. Practicing in a world driven by people seeking immediate relief and thinking in an allopathic way can be very tough. When you choose to become an alternative health care provider, you are going against the grain, trying to do your own small part to make people healthier from the inside out, not the outside in. You are like a soldier, fighting for people to begin to understand that their bodies can heal and repair themselves and must be kept in good order *before* they get sick. Therefore, chiropractors tend to be very passionate about what they do. Most chiropractors can tell you the second they were "called" into their profession. I just seemed to be born into it. I began to wonder if perhaps I chose my profession only in an effort to please my dad.

My doubts grew stronger as I became more miserable. I had a hole in my life, and it was called Lacking Passion. Completely burned out, I started to think of other ways I could make a living. Then, about four years ago, I received an email about a supposedly amazing technique, getting amazing results with, among other conditions, fibromyalgia. Very skeptically, I attended a webinar and listened in disbelief to the results these doctors were reporting. A week later, I attended the seminar. While at that seminar, something woke up inside of me. It was passion. Excitement. Understanding.

When I came back, I taught my first fibromyalgia class to the public. I advertised on the radio and about forty people showed up. I will never forget the first patient I had on my table. Her restless leg was so bad that she had to hook it around the leg of a chair to keep it still during the lecture. She showed all the classic signs of fibromyalgia caused by cervical trauma. When I tested her (as further explained in chapter 5)

I was so nervous that my hands were shaking when I touched her neck. I remember my fingers got wet. Surprised, I looked down. She had tears flowing down her face. I was completely freaked out and asked her if she was OK. When she could finally speak, she said, "No pain. For the first time in twenty-five years *I have no pain.*" After hearing that, her husband started crying too. In that moment, her life changed, and so did mine.

It's been four years since that moment. My life has been completely transformed. These days, I absolutely love helping people who suffer from fibromyalgia. My patients come from all across the world. I have a great passion for this condition. I am a believer, a champion, and a crusader for fibromyalgia. The other day, sitting at DFW airport, I overheard two nurses on their way back from a conference making fun of fibromyalgia. I interrupted them and said, "I couldn't help but overhear you. I am a doctor who also used to not believe in that. May I visit with you?" I do this wherever I go. I have made it my life's work to help people in severe pain, such as fibromyalgia and RSD/CRPS (Reflex Sympathetic Dystrophy, or Central Regional Pain Syndrome), and to educate the public about it.

A few of my patients have told me that had it not been for my intervention, they would have committed suicide. How privileged am I, that I get the chance to change and save lives? It's like throwing a rock in the pond, where the ripple effect goes on beyond your understanding. When people get their lives back, the effects of it are far-reaching. *Everyone* around them is affected. I make it my life's mission to keep my skills and education current and cutting-edge, often ahead of what the masses know. I am constantly learning. My other job, which I charged myself with, is delivering that knowledge to those who need it. I want to make a difference.

I am incredibly blessed. I have found my passion: helping those in chronic, debilitating pain. I can never go back to a life without passion or purpose. In addition, I knew that I could not keep this light that I have discovered under a bucket, so one year ago I sat down and started writing this book. Hopefully, because of it, I will get to touch your life too.

Dr. Katinka

And now, let's begin that journey toward understanding your condition together and get to know the beast (I could insert another *b* word here) known as fibromyalgia.

CHAPTER 1

A BRIEF HISTORY: UNDERSTANDING THE NATURE OF THE BEAST

*I like the dreams of the future better
than the history of the past.*
—*Thomas Jefferson*

*There is no part of my life, upon which
I can look back without pain.*
—*Florence Nightingale*

Isn't the history of fibromyalgia *fascinating?* For most people, probably not so much. Agreed. Let me just say right off the bat that my intention with this book is to help you. It's not to bore you to tears. (Although you do have more time than the average person to read, seeing that people suffering from fibromyalgia sadly don't sleep much.) It's not to use difficult medical terminology, and it's not to write about things that do not really matter to you or your life. It is important to me that this book make a difference to your life, and that every word in it counts. I respect your time.

So why, you may ask, did I start off with a boring thing like the history of fibromyalgia? It is my belief that you arm yourself best by studying the enemy. In your case, the enemy is fibromyalgia. It has changed the quality of your life, reduced the amount of joy you get out of life, and to some extent probably affected every relationship you have. It is your beast that you are battling. Know thy beast. Understand its history and nature so that you can understand yourself. The most important thing that I want you to get from this chapter is that you are not alone. Famous people have known the same pain you know and have suffered from the same symptoms. Now, let's plunge in.

A BRIEF HISTORY

When was fibromyalgia first recognized? For several centuries, muscle pains were known as rheumatism and then as muscular rheumatism. Gowers coined the term fibrositis in 1904. In 1913 in the *British Medical Journal*, a physician by the name of Luff talked about the factors of fibrositis. He noted that the symptoms grew worse when the barometric pressure lowered and rain was approaching. Chances are, if you suffer from fibromyalgia you are probably familiar with this phenomenon (human weather detector, anyone?) It is interesting to me that almost every fibromyalgia patient of mine can tell when it is going to rain, as increased barometric pressure tends to make their symptoms worse and their pain more intense, yet this is one of the symptoms of fibromyalgia not well understood at all. We will finally shed some light on this symptom further on in this book (chapter 5).

The term fibrositis was not changed to fibromyalgia until 1976. The first controlled clinical study with validation of known symptoms and tender points was published in 1981. At first fibromyalgia was thought to be a disease of the muscles and fibrous tissues, which was a logical assumption, since muscle pain seemed to be the main symptom.

However, tests done on the muscles and tissues of FM patients failed to show any actual connection.

Next, researchers theorized that it might be an autoimmune disorder, but actual research could never uncover any disturbance of the immune system, although patients who suffer from fibromyalgia often develop autoimmune conditions (more about this in chapter 6).

Finally, in 1987, the American Medical Association (AMA) recognized fibromyalgia as a real condition. As the twenty-first century approached and technology brought new laboratory testing methods and brain-imaging techniques, researchers were able to identify a sensitization of the central nervous system in fibromyalgia patients. Throughout this book, the central nervous system and its role in fibromyalgia will be explained in detail.

Even though the AMA started recognizing fibromyalgia as a real condition starting in 1987, finding an allopathic doctor who would treat fibromyalgia, much less diagnose it, before 2007, was very challenging. Even though some alternative health care providers treated fibromyalgia long before 2007, most of the medical world as well as the public were largely uninformed about this strange condition, and still debating whether it even existed. Doctors' (mostly pain management doctors') drug of choice to prescribe for fibromyalgia was Oxycontin, adding the high risk of addiction to these patients' problems.

However, in 2007, to the delight of fibromyalgia sufferers as well as advocacy groups, everything changed. Pfizer's medication Lyrica became the first-ever drug approved by the FDA to treat fibromyalgia. Lyrica was originally created to treat diabetic shingles pain, but it showed great promise in relieving the pain of fibromyalgia. During the first nine months of 2007, Pfizer spent $46 million on Lyrica ads. Since that time, the billions of dollars spent advertising Lyrica have brought fibromyalgia into the consciousness of the public as well as the general medical community. (In 2008, Cymbalta followed shortly on Lyrica's heels, bringing even more attention to fibromyalgia.)

Of course, in my opinion, taking Lyrica is a double-edged sword, and choosing to take it may be a difficult decision. Although Lyrica does provide some relief, patients find it to be expensive, with a host of nasty side effects that include dry mouth, headaches, nausea, and last but not least, may cause an annoying weight gain for some.

Today, ongoing research continues to uncover exciting new information about the causes and treatment of FM. Researchers from Georgetown University and the University of Michigan used functional MRI (magnetic resonance imaging) testing and found that when they applied pressure to the thumbnails of a group of fibromyalgia patients, brain activity was activated in twelve areas of the brain compared to only two locations in healthy controls. When the researchers increased thumbnail pressure in the controls, their subjective pain ratings and pain activity also increased, but only eight of the areas of the brain activated were similar to those in the fibromyalgia patients.

So there is the definitive research. It *is* in your head. But it is also real.

YOU ARE NOT ALONE! FAMOUS PEOPLE WHO MAY HAVE SUFFERED FROM FIBROMYALGIA

I, too, have been assigned months of futility, long and weary nights of misery. When I go to bed, I think, 'When will it be morning?' But the night drags on, and I toss till dawn. And now my heart is broken. Depression haunts my days. My weary nights are filled with pain as though something were relentlessly gnawing at my bones.
—Job 7:3–4; 30:16–17

Fibromyalgia, as you probably already know too well, is a horrible condition. It may affect as many as 4 to 5 percent of the population. Its prevalence is similar to that of diabetes or coronary heart disease, yet there's a good chance that the average Joe (or Jane) has never even heard of it.

Unlike these other conditions mentioned above, fibromyalgia is not considered life-threatening. This is probably why it is not more widely understood. Illnesses and conditions that aren't contagious or a significant cause of death rarely stir up enthusiasm in people who don't suffer from them. For this reason, fibromyalgia remains an underdiagnosed disease. But when was it first recognized?

It seems that there is strong evidence through history of people suffering from fibromyalgia-like symptoms. It has been said that Job (from the book of Job) suffered from symptoms that closely resembled the symptoms of fibromyalgia. Even though there is no way to prove this now, anyone who suffers from fibromyalgia will certainly feel a certain kinship with Job, should they carefully read about his history and symptoms.

It is said that Florence Nightingale suffered from fibromyalgia. If you studied her history, you would see how, after she returned from the war in the Crimea where she was faced with deplorable conditions, she took to her bed, often refusing visitors, with invisible ailments and a nameless condition, suffering from profound fatigue. Sadly, she suffered until her death, and her condition was never understood in her own time.

Other famous people who are rumored to may have suffered from fibromyalgia include Charles Darwin, the nineteenth century English naturalist famous for his theory of natural selection, and Frida Kahlo, a Mexican painter, who is said to have suffered fibromyalgia-like symptoms following a bus accident. Her pain is reflected in her art, as many of her most famous paintings depict her body as being tortured by nails and various bindings, her spine replaced by a broken column on the verge of crumbling, or as bedridden.

Another celebrity who suffers from fibromyalgia is the Irish singer Sinead O'Connor, who has said that although she has a "high pain threshold" (common among fibromyalgia sufferers), the fatigue she suffers from has been debilitating and has affected her singing career. Fibromyalgia not only robs people of the opportunity to live the healthy, comfortable life that other people take for granted, but it keeps hundreds of thousands of people from contributing their unique gifts to society, and that affects all of us.

YOUR MOTHER'S MOTHER AND MAYBE YOUR AUNT BETH: DOES FIBROMYALGIA RUN IN FAMILIES?

Throughout the years, I have noticed that fibromyalgia often runs in families. Below are some examples of research that backs this genetic hypothesis up.

- The Swedish Twin Registry reports that there is up to a 15 percent higher chance of one twin developing fibromyalgia if the other twin suffers from it.

- Studies suggested that fibromyalgia segregates within families in an autosomal dominant mode of inheritance. One of them (Pellegrino MJ, Walonis GW, Sommer A: **Familial occurrence of primary fibromyalgia**), showed female preponderance and, in addition, postulated the existence of a latent or precursor stage of the disease characterized by abnormal muscle tension.

- Another study (Stormorken and colleagues Roizenblatt S, Tufik S, Goldenberg J, Pinto LR, Hilario MO, Feldman D: **Juvenile fibromyalgia: clinical and polysomnographic aspects**) was based on data retrieved from questionnaires regarding fibromyalgia symptoms in family members of index patients. According to this study, about two-thirds of the study population reported family clustering.

So what does all this research mean? If you have family members with fibromyalgia, there may be a higher chance of you developing the condition. However, all is not hopeless. The noted scientist Bruce Lipton, PhD, is one of many scientists today proving that we are, in fact, not victims of our genetic material. Dr. Lipton is a well-respected cellular biologist who has done extensive research at Stanford University on the mechanics of genetics and cellular biology.

Most of us were taught that the genetic blueprint we inherited from our parents predetermines our bodies, our personalities, our talents, and even our health. But in the last two decades, Dr. Lipton and other cellular biologists have discovered that, while our genes do not change, the way they are *expressed* may be very much within our control. In layman's terms, this means that even though we may have a higher risk of developing certain conditions or diseases because of our biology, we have a lot of power to *minimize* those risks.

This is good news! Since Dr. Lipton first observed two cells with exactly the same genetic code, in two different petri dishes (different environments), behaving in very different ways, his work has become a foundation for scientific documentation of the mind-body connection. He explains that based on their genetic code, "cells can do a job that contributes to the growth of the organism, its maintenance, and keeping it healthy, or a cell can get into a position of a protection response. Cells need the brain to interpret the world and feed back to them what they should be doing to keep this whole system alive and floating."

According to Dr. Lipton, the true secret to life does not lie within your DNA, but rather within the mechanisms of your cell membrane. Each cell is surrounded by a membrane with receptors attached to it.

Think of them as tiny cell phone towers receiving signals. These receptors pick up signals from their environment, which in turn control how the genes are read inside the cells. In other words, your cells can choose to read or ignore your genetic blueprint depending on the signals they receive from their environment. Simply put, this means that even potentially undesired cell behavior needs a very specific key to unlock it. This key is usually a physical, chemical, or emotional stress. The power to arm your body against this stress lies in your hands.

So, this means that having a "cancer program" or a "fibromyalgia program" in your DNA does not mean you are destined to get cancer or develop fibromyalgia. Isn't that good news? *You* control your environment to a large extent. You control your daily thoughts, your surroundings, your exercise habits, and your diet. You *do* have control over which genes are turned on and turned off. (For more on Dr. Lipton's work, go to www.brucelipton.com.)

The bottom line? Be diligent. Live healthfully. Treat all upper cervical injuries as potentially serious (as described in chapter 5). Don't live in fear of fibromyalgia just because a family member suffers from it, or fear for your child(ren) because you suffer from it. The first step in fighting any enemy is to arm yourself with knowledge.

CHAPTER 2

WHACK-A-MOLE: THE MYSTERIOUS SYMPTOMS YOU MAY NOT ASSOCIATE WITH FIBROMYALGIA

Karma karma karma karma karma chameleon,
You come and go, you come and go...
—*Culture Club*

I wonder if I've been changed in the night? Let me
think. Was I the same when I got up this morning? I
almost think I can remember feeling a little different.
But if I'm not the same, the next question is 'Who
in the world am I?' Ah, that's the great puzzle.
—*Alice in Wonderland*

Let's face it, some people probably think you are kooky and that your symptoms are all in your head. I know it isn't fair; none of these people have walked in your shoes. However, it is part of the unfortunate reality of suffering from fibromyalgia. I will bet that somewhere along the line, you have met a doctor who, although he or she appeared to be sitting there carefully nodding while you were explaining your loooooong list of symptoms, was mentally counting all the ways you seemed nuttier than a Chinese chicken salad.

In my own practice, I have actually had fibromyalgia patients bring in a typed list of their symptoms. Hey, I understand this practice. Most probably, you have had to repeat the same long list thirty-two times or so to different doctors over the years. It gets old. One of your symptoms is having trouble remembering things. You may leave important things off! Why not come prepared? To the average doctor, however, you may as well be wearing a T-shirt reading, "Caution: high-maintenance patient coming through." I am sorry if that offends you. However, my intention throughout this book is to shoot straight from the hip—no coddling, and no mincing words. After all, this can't exactly be news to you. I hear this so often from fibromyalgia patients that I felt it was important to address it.

How do I know this? Well, I happen to have quite a few MDs, chiropractors, osteopaths, and other health care professionals as friends. Add to this all my patients who have told me that this or that doctor "did not believe in fibromyalgia." (Don't let me get started on *that* little nugget, by the way. It makes me angry.) However, I do need to add to this paragraph, reluctantly and apologetically, that I used to agree with those doctors myself, back when I didn't understand fibromyalgia. I have since drastically revised my opinion, and will take this opportunity to humbly say my *mea culpa* and tell you how very wrong I was.

So what gives, you may ask. Why this unfair treatment by the public, as well as your doctors? Well, let me try my best to explain. Not that it makes it OK, but perhaps it will shed some light on the subject.

WHY PEOPLE WITH FIBROMYAGIA ARE DIFFICULT TO TREAT

A lot of doctors have big egos. It's true! We don't mean to. It's just that, to make it through all those tough years of school, you have to have a certain competitive streak in you, an inner grit. We usually choose our profession hoping to help everybody. Somewhere deep inside, we hope that we can. Every. Body. When patients do not respond to care, we get frustrated because we think that we are failing. And, as shameful as it is, when we fail, perhaps subconsciously, sometimes we like to blame the patient. Especially if the condition they suffer from is a chronic one, we are more likely to label patients as "difficult." Let's see why:

First and foremost, by some very unfortunate happenstance, patients with fibromyalgia fit the classic malingering mold. What does this mean? Basically, "malingering" is just a fancy word for faking. All health care professionals are taught to watch out for those patients—those few rotten apples and poor souls who, for whatever reasons, fake their symptoms, ruining it all for the legitimately sick. Let's look at the actual definition of the word:

"Malingering should be suspected when psychological or physical symptoms are accompanied by specific criteria. The first criterion is suspicion of voluntary control of symptoms as demonstrated by one or more indicators, which include bizarre or absurd symptomatology, atypical symptomatic fluctuation consistent with external incentives, or unusual symptomatic response to treatment that cannot otherwise be explained (e.g., paradoxical response to medication)."[1]

That means, in layman's terms, that if your symptoms are shifting all over the place (you may have low back pain one day, pain in your feet the next, and bladder problems on another), doctors are trained to think that you may just be looking for a free ride or attention. You may be thinking that if you wanted attention that badly, you'd just take your clothes off at a local football game and streak across the field. I know. Don't shoot the messenger! For some reason, people often assume fibromyalgia patients just want attention like naughty two-year-olds. Now, add to this the mysterious, ever-changing list of symptoms fibromyalgia patients suffer from. It's tough to diagnose and treat. I like to refer to this phenomenon as "whack-a-mole" in my clinic. Just when you manage to whack one symptom down, another pops up.

In addition, fibromyalgia is a predominantly female condition (although it can absolutely strike men and children). In years past, the medical profession was predominantly male, and women were still thought of as the weaker sex, without enough common sense to even vote. Females presenting with all those mysterious symptoms were often seen as hysterical, difficult, and high-strung. Doctors would prescribe drugs like Valium (and later Prozac) to these women in order to help them be more calm and relaxed. It is only years later that women really found their voice and could protest this treatment.

Of course, once again, the symptoms of fibromyalgia make this condition extremely puzzling and tricky to treat. Let's look at the reasons that may cause your symptoms to appear mysterious. Has the electricity to your house ever shut off? Did you happen to notice that it affected several appliances? You couldn't dry your hair with a hairdryer. You couldn't use the microwave oven. All the lights were off. Did you run around like a mad person, trying to fix each appliance? No! That would be ludicrous and a giant waste of time. Clearly, it was a power problem. You knew that once the power kicked back in, everything would most likely work again.

Think of your nervous system as your electrical system. In your case, it isn't connecting. This is not merely my opinion, but also based on some sound research. One of the lead investigators studying the role of the central nervous system (CNS) in fibromyalgia, Dr. Daniel Clauw, remarked that not only do abnormalities in the brain and central nervous system seem to "spill over" into the body and produce the collection of symptoms we know as fibromyalgia, but there is also evidence that injuries, illnesses, or other major stressors in the body can overwhelm the brain and CNS and cause different symptoms.[2]

More recently, Manuel Martínez-Lavín, MD, and his team at the National Cardiology Institute of Mexico used a special technology known as heart rate variability analysis to demonstrate that the multisystemic symptoms of fibromyalgia (i.e., pain, insomnia, numbness and tingling, migraines, irritable bowel syndrome, etc.) are in fact a result of a dysfunction of the autonomic nervous system (ANS). The automatic system regulates body temperature, blood pressure, and heart rate as well as bowel and bladder tone, and is capable of acting with great rapidity and intensity.[3] In other words, your nervous system very well may be on the fritz, resulting in a lot of the symptoms you suffer from.

ALL THOSE MYSTERIOUS SYMPTOMS

One of the biggest frustrations of working with a fibromyalgia patient, to me, is how their symptoms are mismanaged. For example: fibromyalgia patients often undergo needless surgeries. Let's use arthroscopic surgery of the knee as an example. Many fibromyalgia patients will develop knee problems such as arthritis-like pain and decreased range of motion or weakness. These symptoms are often much worse when it is cold or when bad weather passes through. Very few doctors link these symptoms to fibromyalgia. Even if they do, however, knee surgery is still often performed.

In 2002, J. Bruce Moseley, currently a clinical associate professor at the Baylor Sports Medicine Institute in House, headed a randomized study to find out exactly how effective knee arthroscopies were. During this study, it was found that osteoarthritis patients, prime candidates for arthroscopy, fared no better than patients who received a sham surgery.[4] However, knee arthroscopy today remains among the top ten outpatient procedures, with more than six hundred and fifty thousand surgeries performed yearly.

Let's refer back to the electricity/appliance analogy. If the electricity to the toaster is shut off, should you fix or replace the toaster? Yet most doctors look at large joint pain as a local problem—a toaster problem, if you will. I have had several patients who assured me that no, their problem is an *actual* anatomical problem confirmed by MRI. "My doctor said my knee is bone on bone and my only hope is knee replacement surgery." Then, after addressing the problem within their central nervous system, their knee pain mysteriously disappeared. What gives? Is it possible that even though the joint was abnormal, this was merely a *symptom* of another problem, and not the actual cause of the pain? My clinical experience certainly taught me that this is often the case. I am not saying that knee surgery should *never* be the answer. I am just saying that invasive and dangerous surgery should not be one of the *first* answers. The problem is that most patients, and also doctors for that matter, were not taught to link central nervous system malfunction to joint pain.

Now is a good time to bring up a very important point. Who is responsible for your health? You are. Who cares most about your health? You do. It is *your* responsibility to make sense of your symptoms—to not only *understand* them, but to understand what is causing them. This goes for all aspects of your health. If your doctor prescribes a medication, it is your responsibility to research the side effects of that specific medication. Isn't that what Google is for? With the Internet available these days, this is not a difficult thing to do. For example, this way, you can hear from tens of thousands of other patients taking the same medication, not just what the drug company or FDA told your doctor.

Never, ever trust other people with your health blindly. You *must* be your own best advocate. Imagine handing your wedding ring to your doctor. "Oh, here, doc. Can you keep this for me over the weekend?" You would never do that, right? It is too valuable a possession.

Yet we frequently hand our bodies to our doctors lock, stock, and barrel, fully trusting that it will all somehow be OK. How much more precious is your health than your wedding ring?

The next step to understanding your own condition is understanding all the symptoms that may be associated with it. The symptoms of fibromyalgia are confusing at best. Most of the websites out there, in my opinion, do not give a complete list of symptoms. For your convenience, I will list the symptoms by body region. This list was assimilated based on listening to thousands of fibromyalgia patients, rather than on specific research. We have found that the same symptoms tend to crop up over and over. First, let's take a look at the most common way fibromyalgia is diagnosed by doctors.

THE TENDER POINTS

The most well-known way fibromyalgia is usually diagnosed is by the doctor locating and identifying specific tender points in the fibromyalgia patient. There are eighteen tender points important for the diagnosis of fibromyalgia (see image below). These tender points are located in specific spots on your body. To get a medical diagnosis of fibromyalgia, eleven of the eighteen tender points must be painful when lightly pressed. Please note that if you take pain medication prior to the exam, it could produce a false negative result.

In addition to this exam, doctors will usually base their diagnosis on a careful history and a list of all of your symptoms. However, in my experience, a lot of patients suffering from fibromyalgia (and even doctors) still experience confusion about which of their symptoms are normal and which are abnormal. Below, I will attempt to shed some light on those.

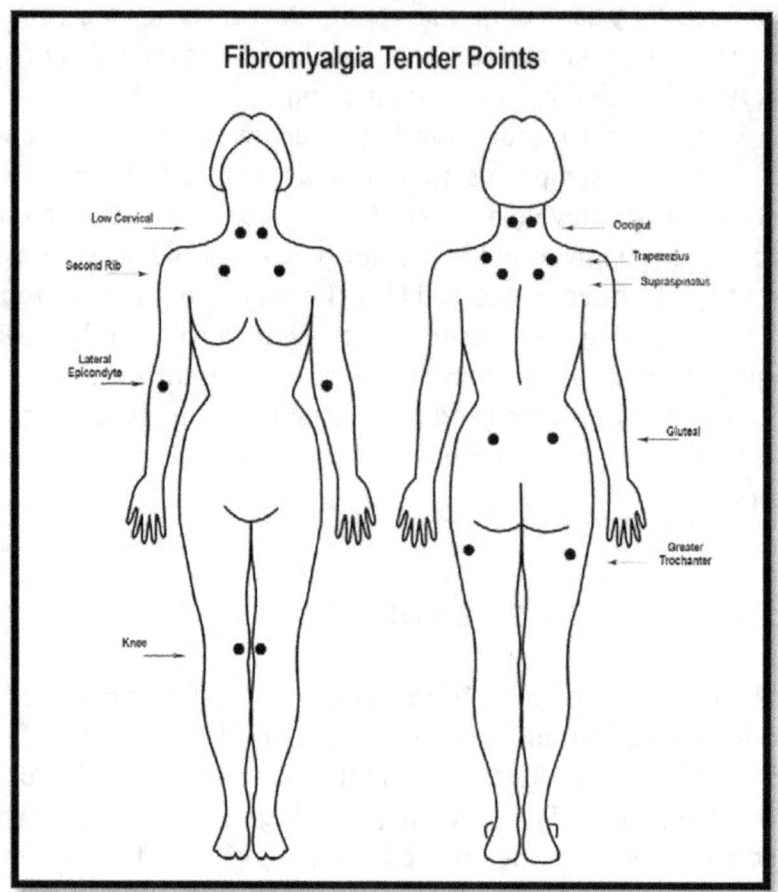

ALL THE OTHER SYMPTOMS

YOUR CRANIAL NERVES:
THE FRONT DOOR TO YOUR NERVOUS SYSTEM

The cranial nerves are twelve pairs of nerves on the ventral (bottom) surface of the brain. These nerves control a lot of important things, and their purpose is mainly to connect you with the world around your body. Think of these nerves as your nervous system's front door to the world. These nerves allow you to hear, see, taste, and smell. Some of these nerves bring information from the sense organs to the brain. Some control muscles; others are connected to glands or internal organs such as the heart and lungs. One of the main functions of these nerves, in our caveman days and still today, is to perceive danger. We do this through our sensory nervous system. The cranial nerves in almost every fibromyalgia patient show abnormalities. Here is how the malfunction of these important nerves may affect you:

- Taste loss

- Speech disturbances, which can be so severe that it sounds as if you have suffered from a stroke

- Balance loss

- A feeling of fullness in your ears

- Eye pain

- Ever-changing eyesight and visual disturbances (if you are reading this book on an e-reader and had to change the font, this may be affecting you)

- Light sensitivity

- Blurred vision

- Feelings of disorientation, especially when going to a store like Costco or Sam's Club (these stores have large open spaces with no horizons, lots of visual stimulation, and the need for you to focus)

- Feelings of disorientation while in an elevator

- Fainting

- Lightheadedness

- Nausea

- Carsickness or disorientation while riding in a car, especially when you look at strobe lights like the ones that emergency vehicles use

- Dizziness

- Ears ringing

- Ears buzzing

- Intolerance to loud sounds, such as a baby crying

- Hearing loss

- Inability to tolerate large crowds

- One-sided facial pain

- Pain in your teeth

- Jaw pain

- Difficulty swallowing

YOUR ACHY HEAD AND NECK

The cervical spine (neck) and any history of injuries to this area that you may have are so crucial that we will devote an entire chapter to them later. For now, let's just focus on your actual symptoms.

- Headaches

- Migraines

- One-sided headaches

- One-sided migraines

- Pain in back of head or base of skull

- Pain in either temple

- "Heavy" head

- Memory loss

- Neck pain

- Pain when moving your neck

- Stiff neck

- Muscle spasm

- Neck "grinds" or "pops"

- Difficulty in moving neck

- Nerves feel "pinched"

- Disc problems

- TMJ (temporomandibular joint) pain and problems

- Pain in the face (trigeminal neuralgia)

- Clenching your teeth at night

- Teeth grinding

- Pain that radiates into your teeth

BURDEN ON YOUR SHOULDERS

- Shoulder pain

- Rotator cuff problems

- Pain across your shoulders

- Tense or "hard" upper back and shoulder muscles, or what I refer to as "concrete shoulders" in my office

- Cannot lift arm above shoulder level

- Nerve pain or numbness in either (or both) shoulder(s)

- Tension in either (or both) shoulder(s)

- Pain in either (or both) arm(s)

- Forearm pain

- Finger pain

- Cold hands

- Swelling in either (or both) hand(s)

- Pain in either (or both) wrist(s)

- Pain in either (or both) hand(s)

- Arthritis in fingers

- Weak grip, for example when opening bottles

- Dropping things a lot

- Tingling in any part of the upper extremities

MID-BACK AND CHEST

- Mid-back pain

- Pain when you wear a bra

- Pain between shoulder blades

- Mid-back spasms

- Pain when you get a massage

- Chest pain

- Pain in your breastbone

- Pain that feels like it's coming from your heart

- Shortness of breath

- Pain in your ribs (in the front or back)

- Difficulty breathing

LOW BACK

- Low back pain

- Muscle spasms

- Stiff low back

- Arthritis

- Disc problems, such as herniated discs

- Arthritis in the lower back

- Decreased movement of the lower back

ABDOMEN

(When you are passing more gas than a pregnant woman expecting triplets)

- Gas

- Nausea

- Constipation

- Diarrhea

- Crohn's disease

- Irritable bowel syndrome (IBS)

- Heartburn

- Gluten intolerance/allergies

- Menstrual pain

- Cramping

- Irregularity

- Heavy cycles

- Abdominal pain

- Irritated stomach

- Abnormal pap smears

- Ovarian cysts

- Infertility

HIPS/LEGS/FEET

(Honey, no one is running a marathon around here anytime soon.)

- Pain in buttocks

- Pain in one or both hips

- Pain in one or both legs

- Knee pain/problems (even diagnosed arthritis)

- Pain in one or both ankles

- Pain in one or both feet

- Feeling of walking on "broken glass"

- Numbness in either (or both) leg(s)

- Numbness in either (or both) foot (feet)

- Numb toes

- Cold feet (not the kind you get before getting married)

- Burning in either foot

- Cramps in your legs or feet

- Swollen ankles

- Swollen feet

- Pain in toes

- Restless legs

- "Creepy-crawly" feeling in legs at night

ALL THE OTHER ICKY SYMPTOMS

- Suicidal feelings

- Depression

- Anxiety

- Panic attacks

- Nervousness

- Irritability

- Loss of periods of time

- Memory loss

- Fogginess

- Forgetfulness

- Pain during or after exercise

- Pain when rain is coming or the weather is changing

- Intolerance to heat

- Intolerance to cold

- Intolerance to the wind

- Skin rashes

- Hair loss

- Bladder pain

- Urinary incontinence

- Feeling of constant fullness in the bladder

- Pain upon urination

- Pain during sexual intercourse or decreased libido

- "Creepy-crawly" feelings all over, or "lightning bolts" of pain

- Insomnia

- Waking up a lot

- Sleep apnea

- Intense, relentless fatigue (when you don't care if the house burns down to the ground around you—you can't get off your couch)

- Vaginal pain/burning

We are well aware that if you don't personally suffer from fibromyalgia, you may look at this list and think, "Doesn't that include pretty much everybody?" That is *exactly* the problem that fibromyalgia patients face. Since the list of symptoms they suffer from is so lengthy and affects the entire body, it often rouses suspicion in doctors and the public alike. It doesn't help that the symptoms come and go and can change from one area of the body to another, just depending on the day.

However, if you keep in mind that the central nervous system affects every single part of the body, it is not difficult to understand why this is the case. Remember our power failure example from earlier? Furthermore, keep in mind that even though most of us will have a few of these symptoms at some point in life, fibromyalgia patients suffer from *many* of the symptoms we listed all at once, not just a few every now and then.

We hope that this chapter helped you to make a bit of sense of all your mysterious symptoms. That being said, you really have to get to know your own body. If any symptoms are new, out of the ordinary, or alarming, do not hesitate to see your doctor. It is entirely possible for you to develop a symptom that signals that something else is wrong with your health. Do not make the mistake of brushing *all* of your symptoms under the fibromyalgia rug. Most importantly, do not allow your doctor to do this, either. When it comes to your health, always, always follow your gut and be diligent.

CHAPTER 3

YOU LOOK FINE TO ME: HOW TO EDUCATE THOSE AROUND YOU

Absence from those we love is self from self—a deadly banishment.
—*William Shakespeare*

Have compassion for everyone you meet even if they don't want it. What seems conceit, bad manners, or cynicism is always a sign of things no ears have heard, no eyes have seen. You do not know what wars are going on down there where the spirit meets the bone.
—*Miller Williams (American poet)*

'It doesn't happen all at once,' said the Skin Horse. 'You become. It takes a long time. That's why it doesn't happen often to people who break easily, or have sharp edges, or who have to be carefully kept. Generally, by the time you are Real, most of your hair has been loved off, and your eyes drop out and you get loose in the joints and very shabby. But these things don't matter at all, because once you are Real you can't be ugly, except to people who don't understand.'
—*Margery Williams, The Velveteen Rabbit*

One of the toughest things about suffering from fibromyalgia, in my opinion, is living in a fibro-unfriendly world. The number one complaint we hear from people with this condition, besides the obvious discomfort they suffer from, is that they sometimes feel belittled, alone, and even ridiculed. We have explained what we believe lies behind this trend. However, we have decided to devote an entire chapter just to ways of coping with this. Coping is better than complaining about how things are or should be. It is so much easier to swim with the current, rather than fight against it. As the old saying goes, it is better to light a single candle than to curse the darkness.

WHAT TO TELL YOUR FAMILY

If you think of fibromyalgia as a war, think of your family as your fellow soldiers. They are the ones who have, or should have, your back. Unfortunately, fibromyalgia patients often feel alone in their own homes. Even the most supportive family members will sometimes get sick and tired of your being sick and tired. The main reason that your family may not be as supportive as you would like them to be is lack of understanding. The German poet Goethe said, "Everyone hears only what he understands." It is your job to help your family understand your condition. In order to do this, you must understand your own condition and not merely manage its symptoms.

Start by educating yourself about each symptom. This book will help to explain many of the symptoms you suffer from. For example: the fibromyalgia patient's friends and family often experience the patient's fatigue as laziness or lack of enthusiasm. The fact that you often do not have the energy to participate in activities may cause them frustration. When your family understands that fatigue is a real physical symptom with a very real cause, there is a good possibility that they will act more tolerant. If not, you can only try your best. Do not let feelings of guilt, inadequacy, and shame rule your life. When you find yourself feeling these things, pretend for a moment that you suffer from another condition or illness, such as breast cancer. Then ask yourself: would I be feeling guilty if my symptoms had a different label? All you can do in every situation is your best.

Part of my education process with patients consists of sitting down with them and asking them what their three highest values are in life. Is it family? Is it religion? Most people rate their spiritual life as one, their family as two, and their career as three. I then usually gently point out to the patient that unless they have their health, they can't fully function in any of these areas. If your ill health causes your body to expire or, in a less extreme case, forces you to become bedridden, it becomes much more difficult to honor those values. If your *quality* of life severely declines, the quantity often ceases to matter as much.

It is my belief that your health should always be rated above everything else, even when it comes to the needs of your children. Does this seem selfish? Allow me to explain. If you have ever traveled with your child on an airplane, the flight crew probably told you before your flight took off that in case of an emergency, you were to put your own oxygen mask on first and only *then* put on your child's. The concept is simple. You cannot serve anything or anyone unless you can function.

Your health is your most precious possession. You should look after it as such, *especially* if you already face challenges and your health is somewhat fragile. It is not altruistic or selfless to push your body harder than you should in order to serve others. People who suffer from fibromyalgia, in an effort not to disappoint those they love, often push their bodies to perform even though they are hurting and bone-tired. While commendable and understandable, doing this is actually unwise and may ultimately hurt the very people you love. If you had a broken leg, you wouldn't walk on it, would you? Forcing your body to exercise, to perform, and to push through when you hurt may do more damage than good.

I understand that you may have a job, and probably a family that needs meals to be put on the table and bills to be paid. Life is going on around you, and you must participate in it to some extent. However, I do not appreciate when doctors and well-meaning people tell fibromyalgia patients to try and exercise harder, to do more. You have to respect the terrific burden your body is already under. Coddle it, feed it good quality food, and rest when you can.

IF YOU HAVE YOUNG CHILDREN

As the mother of a five-year-old boy, I find it particularly sad to hear a patient talking about the fact that he or she cannot be the mother, father, or grandparent the person wants to be to his or her children or grandchildren. The one overriding emotion they all seem to deal with in abundance is guilt. They feel guilt because they have to lie down a lot. They feel guilt over hurting all the time, guilt that they can't enjoy family activities with their loved ones. They experience tremendous guilt over the fact that they cannot be the parent or grandparent they wish to be—fully active, present, and happy all around.

In chapter 14, you will read Noreen's story. Noreen was a very successful ER nurse before she became ill with fibromyalgia, twenty-five years before she became my patient. We will cover her story in detail, since it is an amazing one of hope and recovery. The part I want to tell you about now happened in about her seventh week of care. Her twenty-year-old daughter Becca was visiting from Texas and came in with her mom to meet me. (At this stage, Noreen was about 75 percent symptom-free.) Noreen had suffered from fibromyalgia throughout her daughter's life. Becca was naturally shy, but she walked up to me that day and hugged me and said something I will never forget: "Thank you for giving me my mom back. I have never met her. This woman is not the same woman who raised me." I had tears in my eyes. That moment strengthened me in my purpose to help other people like Becca get their loved ones back.

The sad truth is that your child might not know or remember the "you" you were before you became sick. However, try to remember that we are bound to feel guilty when we have children. There will always be *something* we think we could be doing better. So just be the best parent that you can be. You did not choose to be sick. You don't have to be perfect as long as you love your child. Nobody can do that better than you. I bet that one day, when your child is an adult and looks back, they would still choose to have had you around, exhausted and in pain, rather than not having had you around at all.

Just do the best you can. Surround yourself with a strong support network that can pick up the slack where you fall short sometimes. Someone who can tolerate that giant mouse and the yelling cheerleaders at Chuck E. Cheese. Someone who can pick up some loose ends. You don't have to be a perfect healthy parent. What matters is being there at night to tuck them in and tell them you love them. Explain that sometimes you don't feel well, but that everything is going to be OK, that you are doing your best, and that you love them and always will.

If you have a significant other, understand that if your roles were reversed, you would be the primary practical caregiver. Let them be that, and you focus on just doing the best you can while still being gentle with your sick body. Never give up looking for help, because people *have* gotten better. This condition can be managed. Fight for your children or grandchildren and for yourself, but remember that they love you just the way you are while you are doing it. When people offer to help you, accept help. Your condition is every bit as real as cancer. You deserve support where and when you can get it. Do not try to be a superhero.

IF YOU HAVE GRANDCHILDREN

When grandparents suffer from fibromyalgia, they often experience tremendous guilt. There is a certain expectation in modern society that a grandma or grandpa should supply carefree happiness and unconditional love. Often, in households where both parents are working, the grandparent will step in to lighten the burden of care-giving on the parents and to babysit when the parents are away. In your case, this may be a lot to ask, leading to tremendous guilt for the grandparent whose body prevents them from fulfilling this role.

You have to understand that you did not choose your condition. You did not choose this life of fatigue and pain. Often, my patients who are grandparents will hide their pain from their family in the fear that they will not get to spend time with their grandchildren. So many times have I heard grandparents express sorrow that they cannot pick up a grandchild due to their pain.

I once treated a grandmother who was less than honest with her son about how bad she felt so that he would still let her babysit her small two- and four-year-old grandsons once a week. After doing so, she would be in bed for two days. She was too scared to reveal this to him, petrified that he would think she didn't want to spend time with them and that she would lose her opportunity to do so. (Sadly, he was less than understanding when it came to her health.) I strongly urged her to stop this and to only take them for two hours at a time while undergoing treatment. She listened to me and devoted a few months to recovering while going through my treatment. Today, she can watch her grandchildren for days at a time with no piper to pay afterward.

It is important that you remember that you don't have to be the perfect grandparent. You just have to love your grandchild(ren) when and how you can. This love can be showed in many shapes and forms. You can love them even when you are hurting. Do not focus on the loss of the things you can't do with them and the things you wish you could. Focus on what you *can* do and do that as best you can. Make sure that you educate your children on the ins and outs of your condition once they are old enough to understand. Do not hesitate to say no to babysitting your grandchildren when you are in a lot of pain. This does not indicate your failure as a grandparent.

It helps to see your body as a vessel of the love you have to give. You *have* to stay as healthy as you can so that your body will allow you to do the things you enjoy: to give more, to love longer, to have more time with those you love. Every choice you make in favor of your health is a deposit into your health account. It is this account you will draw from to give to your grandchildren. When that account is empty, you will have nothing left to give. Rudolph Giuliani one said, "What children need most are the essentials that grandparents provide in abundance. They give unconditional love, kindness, patience, humor, comfort, and lessons in life. And, most importantly, cookies." Give these when you can, and be kind to yourself when you can't.

WHEN FIBROMYALGIA JOINS YOUR MARRIAGE OR RELATIONSHIP: THE NOT-SO-FUN THREESOME

When I start what I consider to be a healing journey with a new fibromyalgia patient, I always insist on meeting with their spouse or significant other. I do this for many reasons, but foremost, I consider it of utmost importance to educate the spouse or significant other about what their loved one faces daily. I encourage every person with a loved one who suffers from fibromyalgia, even if you read nothing else, to read "The Spoon Theory" by Christine Miserandino (found at http://www.butyoudontlooksick.com/wpress/articles/written-by-christine/the-spoon-theory/).

She does a brilliant job of explaining to someone who isn't sick what it's like to live with daily, unrelenting chronic pain. I don't want to explain it here in too much detail, but in short, she compares every daily task the fibromyalgia patient faces with a spoonful of energy. For example, waking up on time, getting out of bed, and taking a shower will equal one spoon. Some mornings you wake up with an allowance of twelve spoons of energy, some mornings with only three.

At the end of the day, you may have no spoons left over to hand to your loved ones.

Spouses or partners of fibromyalgia patients tend to fall into roughly three different categories:

- There is the loving, supportive spouse or partner. I can usually recognize these by the sheer fact that they are there in my office with the sick spouse or partner for the very first visit. They take over the housework and they tend to be concerned, loving, and involved in their spouse's condition.

- The second kind of spouse or partner may have been supportive at first, but is fatigued. They are tired of being the primary breadwinner/parent/caretaker. They have been to many doctors' visits with their spouse or partner and have become disillusioned and perhaps tired of spending money.

- The third kind of spouse or partner is hostile, frustrated, and completely unsupportive. They may refer to their spouse or partner as lazy, looking for attention, or a hypochondriac. They usually will not accompany the patient to their doctor's visit. If they are the sole breadwinner, they may even refuse to pay for the patient's medical care, since it is not a "real" condition in their opinion. If the spouse is female, she may be frustrated because her husband is unable to earn an income. If the spouse or partner is male, they may be tired of their wife or partner complaining—bitter about their inability to earn a living or help around the house and cook dinners. Frequently, they may also be fed up by their partner's inability or unwillingness to have sex, which does little to help their already strained relationship.

A couple of years ago a patient named Sarah was referred to me by her neurosurgeon. Her husband, a corporate attorney, came with her, but obviously not to support her. He was busy with his Blackberry during our entire consultation and was overtly hostile. Finally, impatiently, he leaned over and told me with visible venom that his wife was "worthless" and that her fibromyalgia was "in her head." My heart went out to her as I watched her shrink down in her chair. They left that day, never to come back. To this day, my interaction with this couple haunts me. She seemed utterly alone, miserable, and scared.

I believe that any health crisis, but especially a chronic condition, will test a marriage or relationship. If there are cracks or weaknesses prior to the condition or illness, they may be widened to chasms or canyons. In a sense, suffering from fibromyalgia may be your relationship's ultimate litmus test. Can it survive through sickness and health? People will stay in bad relationships for all sorts of reasons—fear of financial ruin, children, or fear of change. Whatever you do, do not stay because you think that you deserve to be treated badly since you are a burden. Ask yourself this question: If your husband, wife, or partner were chronically ill, would you support him or her? If the answer is yes, know that you deserve no less. You did not choose this condition.

THE OTHER SIDE: LIVING WITH SOMEONE WHO SUFFERS FROM FIBROMYALGIA

While it is true that the person who suffers from fibromyalgia suffers greatly, I would be remiss to not address the other side. For every person who suffers from fibromyalgia, there is usually a partner or loved one(s) suffering right along with him or her. As mentioned above, understanding will bring tolerance. However, that goes both ways. It helps to see both viewpoints. If you are the partner, spouse, child, friend, or sibling of a person who suffers from fibromyalgia, I want to acknowledge your hardships, your suffering, and your dedication. If you are in a relationship or marriage with someone who suffers from fibromyalgia, I also want to address some of the specific challenges you may be facing as a couple.

When your partner is sick or suffers from a lack of energy, many of the household chores will now fall on your shoulders. Cooking, doing laundry, shopping, taking care of pets, doing homework with the kids, and cleaning now become partially (or wholly) your responsibility. This is extra difficult if your partner is unable to work. I believe in only sweating the small things in life. Therefore, it is important that you, as a couple or family, find a new way of doing things. It doesn't really matter if the laundry doesn't get done every day. Please appreciate the tremendous obstacles you both face and tackle what is most important first. If it is within your means financially, hire someone to clean and mow the lawn. Organize all your activities from high priority to low priority. If possible, farm out the low ones.

As a sick person's caregiver, it is important that you find a place to charge your own battery. This may appear in the form of support from your family and friends or in the form of actual support groups for spouses of those who are suffering from chronic illness or for those who need spiritual support of any kind. Just because your partner is suffering does not mean that you cannot still enjoy life. I would like to refer to the oxygen mask example earlier in this chapter. If the plane is in trouble, you must administer oxygen to yourself first so that you can assist others. Make sure that you take time by yourself to replenish *you*. This way you will have more to give. Make sure that you become an expert on what your partner is suffering from. This way you can help to explain their symptoms, lack of energy, and frequent lack of participation in family activities.

When a person suffers from fibromyalgia, their libido may be greatly suppressed. This may be due to pain, medication, lack of sleep, or nervous system interference. Do not take this personally. It does not indicate a lack of love from them. Imagine having the flu every day, for this is roughly how your partner feels. Would you feel frisky? Focus on the better days and agree to enjoy those together to the max. There are still many good memories to be made by the both of you. Fibromyalgia can't take this away from you.

Do not feel guilty when you are frustrated, lonely, or angry. Feelings like these are natural and to be expected in your circumstances. You do not have to be a Stepford wife, husband, or partner at all times. Just do the best you can under the circumstances. Educate the friends and family that surround your relationship so that they may form a circle of love around you both. Lean on them. Take weekends by yourself. Go recharge.

YOUR BOSS AND COWORKERS

Let's get back to you, the person suffering from fibromyalgia. Make sure that you can physically tolerate your job. If your health continues to decline because of it, you should seriously consider changing it to something less strenuous. While it is unfair to be discriminated against by your boss because of your ill health, it is just as unfair to continue to hold a position that you can no longer fulfill due to your ill health. It is not fair to your body, either.

I believe that, unfortunately, discrimination against patients who suffer from fibromyalgia is still very common in the workplace. Therefore, if it is possible for you to fulfill your duties, I would advise you to not discuss your condition too openly at work. I know that my opinion may be somewhat controversial, but as always, I will shoot straight from the hip. Nobody at work wants to hear about your symptoms day in and day out. Your personal health or lack thereof falls under the category of too much information (TMI). At work, you want to seem as capable and "together" as you can possibly be.

While some bosses may be very tolerant and understanding, it is unfortunately true that most will see your condition as a weakness and potential obstacle. Hence my advice to keep your condition somewhat private in the workplace. I am not saying that you should hide it, but don't talk about it around the water cooler too much. See it as a handicap. Yes, you have it. Yes, sometimes it will affect you. Yes, you can deal with it, and you shouldn't be discriminated against because of it. However, I have a personal belief that when it comes to your professional life, you should never show your underbelly.

THE DOCTOR WHO DOESN'T BELIEVE IN FIBROMYALGIA

Don't get me started. Let's keep it short and sweet. The simple solution? Fire this doctor. Seriously. There is such overwhelming scientific evidence today that fibromyalgia does exist that this is not acceptable treatment from the person who is supposed to coach you, support you, and manage your condition. Always remember, your doctor works for *you*. Essentially, you employ them. There are wonderful, compassionate doctors out there who *do* believe that your pain is real. Find yourself a better doctor. If you don't have one locally, I believe a good doctor is worth traveling for. Whatever you do, do not allow any health care provider to make you feel crazy or bad about yourself or to make you doubt what you know is real. Your doctor is the one person who *must* understand your condition and if not show compassion, at least have an understanding of what you are going through.

I have a patient (let's call her Miss Jones) who suffers from lupus. Even though she is fairly young (twenty-six), she is feisty and assertive and completely in control of her case management. I don't think she has ever met a doctor who intimidates her. She has a whole team of them since she suffers from kidney failure and other serious symptoms. Miss Jones told me that she decided early on that it is essential that she likes her doctors and that they be compassionate and understanding of what she is going through. She has ruthlessly and without abandon fired every doctor who showed the smallest sign of carelessness, arrogance, indifference, or incompetence.

Today, she says that although it took her years and ruffling many feathers along the way, she considers her team of doctors invaluable. She, in turn, is a very dedicated patient. She never misses an appointment, and she follows my care plan to a T. Oh, and last but not least, she bakes fabulous cupcakes for my support staff and me.

Think of your team of doctors as a team of NASCAR mechanics. They need to understand your condition. They need to stay open-minded and also be able to think outside the box. They need to communicate with each other and, most importantly, they need to *care about you*. Health care is a consumer's market, and doctors who do not meet your standards should not be allowed to keep your business.

HOW TO BE A GOOD PATIENT

Through my years of working with people, I have worked with quite a few difficult patients. Much as with everything else in life, if *every* health care professional you encounter seems rude and incompetent, there may come a time when you ought to do a bit of self-examining. It's possible, just possible, that you, as the common denominator, might be the bad apple. Hard to conceive of, I know, but self-examination is sometimes crucial, though it is not for the faint of heart.

I try very hard to really love every one of my patients. When they hire me as their doctor, I consider that to be almost a sacred contract. They hand me money and trust me with their bodies. In return, I promise to provide the best, most up-to-date, and most cutting-edge care that I can. I try my best to not bring any personal stress to work. However, I must confess, I have had those few patients whom I just dread seeing. I once walked into my waiting room only to turn on my heel and go hide in my office. When my assistant came to get me out with a question on her face, all I could muster was "I don't wanna! Please don't make me!" The patient in question (may I call her the culprit?) resembled Shirley MacLaine's "Ouiser" from Steel Magnolias. Not only did she often not show up for her appointments and complain loudly that I had never helped her a bit and was basically worthless (all of which I was still willing to overlook), but she was fond of patting my stomach in front of other patients and cheerfully asking me when the baby was due (I wasn't pregnant at the time). This happened at least five times.

I tell this story to drive the following concept home: your doctor is not the enemy. Most of us have our hearts in the right place. It is a fact that working in health care today, especially with the chronically ill, can be a tough job at times. You want your doctors to *like* you when possible. This will make your life a lot easier. Therefore, we ought to discuss what we consider to be the qualities that turn people into bad patients. Let's call it the "do" and the "do not" list:

Do not be late for your appointments. Do pay your bills in a timely manner or make other arrangements if you can't, which do not include dodging your doctor's account manager's phone calls. Most doctors have families and high overheads and are, contrary to common beliefs, not stinking rich, and will be willing to work out a payment plan with you. Do cancel your appointment with more than forty-eight hours' notice when possible. Please be polite, even if you are hurting. Being in pain does not excuse rudeness. Please do not drown your doctor with complaints. This does *not* mean that you should not let them know about what is hurting you. However, there is a fine line between providing information and whining.

If you have a great doctor, make sure to refer other patients to him or her. We always appreciate your vote of confidence. Last but not least, we greatly appreciate when you express gratitude. This may be verbally, or through small gestures. (See Miss Jones's cupcakes above.) I also personally love when a patient celebrates small victories. Overall, I guess you can sum it up as a general attitude of seeing the glass as half full rather than empty. My dad is fond of telling his patients, "What you focus on will expand. If your entire body hurts today, but your pinkie doesn't, be grateful for that pain-free pinkie."

PEOPLE WHO ASK YOU HOW YOU ARE DOING

Once people know that you frequently don't feel well, chances are that they will ask you how you feel all the time. While they usually mean well, this can be extremely annoying. Do not let this become a big obstacle for you. People with fibromyalgia sometimes struggle with this. They don't want to be perceived as "complainers" or "hypochondriacs." If the person is a casual acquaintance, keep it brief but honest. "I am hurting, but it's OK. How are you?" Or you can try, "Well, fibro is kind of a chronic thing, so I have good days and bad days. Today is an OK day. How is your newest grandbaby?" Bring it back around to them. If you sense that they really care and you are closer to them, you can briefly tell them how you feel. It is OK to share that you are hurting. If the person cares about you and is interested, you deserve to honestly tell them how you feel. Fibromyalgia patients have taught themselves, consciously or subconsciously, to wear a mask for the outside world. While this is understandable, it is hardly fair to you.

Speaking of masks:

> *The average person tells four lies a day or one thousand four hundred and sixty a year; a total of eighty-seven thousand six hundred by the age of sixty. And the most common lie is: 'I'm fine.'*
> *—Unknown*

When a fibromyalgia patient starts care in my clinic, I teach them to communicate the severity of their pain on a scale of one to ten. It's called the McGill pain scale, where ten is the worst pain they have ever had and zero equals no pain. Invariably, I get great resistance from the fibro patient at first. They have trained themselves to disassociate from their pain, to minimize it. It is like the pain is happening on a movie screen to someone else. They refuse to acknowledge it, describe it, or dwell on it.

I also believe that the human body is capable of forming the equivalent of a callus when it comes to pain. It learns to numb it down and, in a sense, sequester it and ignore it subconsciously. While the average healthy patient will rate a migraine as a ten on the pain scale, a fibromyalgia patient will invariably rate it as a five or six. Patients who suffer from fibromyalgia will often tell you that they have a very high pain tolerance. They almost wear it like a badge of honor. While this is a common symptom among fibromyalgia patients, it is actually a sign of poor neurological health.

The first step of neurological recovery in fibromyalgia, in my experience, is feeling pain in a normal fashion. This is a sign that your body is returning to normal and not merely surviving, because the nervous system can now acknowledge the injury and address it. Think of it as a crying baby. Babies cry not to annoy us, but to let us know that they need attention of some kind. If you learn to "tune out" the baby, it may be more comfortable for you, but not necessarily a good thing for said baby.

"BUT YOU DON'T LOOK SICK" AND THE OTHER STUPID THINGS PEOPLE MAY SAY TO YOU

Unfortunately, you or your loved ones suffer from a condition that many people have a strong opinion about. The world seems to be divided into three groups: Those who don't know much about fibromyalgia, those who don't believe it is a real condition, and those who do.

I have in recent years turned into a fierce defender of people who suffer from fibromyalgia, and when I hear people making ignorant comments about it, it can really rile me up. I try to stay patient and use the opportunity to educate those people rather than berate. Usually, that goes something like this, "Really? I understand. I actually used to be a doctor who really didn't believe in it either, but since then, I've had my eyes opened for me. I found out that it is a real thing and that people usually can, and want to, recover from it."

As a result of all the feelings the word "fibromyalgia" conjures up, you may deal with a myriad of daily annoyances as you navigate your way through the world. I am of the firm belief that as we give compassion, compassion will be given to us in return. Therefore, I suggest that your handle hurtful comments or questions with humor, and maintain an attitude of tolerance and forgiveness with which to handle all ignorant or insensitive comments. Most people do not mean to be hurtful, but are simply uninformed. Unless they are related to you or a close friend, it is not their responsibility to understand the ins and outs of your condition.

When people tell you that you look healthy, thank them. At least you don't look on the outside like you feel on the inside. If they give you unsolicited advice, thank them. They mean well. If they tell you they don't believe in fibromyalgia, handle it with humor. One of my favorite responses to this comment is, "Oh, is it a religion now? I didn't know!" Do not let the world's ignorance drag you down.

Remember, you start your day with a limited amount of energy. Let's pretend that every morning, a healthy person wakes up with the equivalent of a hundred dollars' worth of energy units. Every action you take that day, every thought you think, every emotion you feel will cost a certain amount of energy. Normal people have enough energy units (or energy "dollars") to spend on anger, annoyance, and other negative emotions. You start *your* day on a painfully low budget. You cannot afford to waste your precious energy units on one thing that does not positively benefit your health. Positive feelings will deposit energy into your account, and negative energy will withdraw from it.

CHAPTER 4

HOW DID YOU GET SICK?

> *Cause and effect, means and ends, seed and fruit cannot be severed; for the effect already blooms in the cause, the end preexists in the means, the fruit in the seed.*
> —Ralph Waldo Emerson

> *The present contains nothing more than the past, and what is found in the effect is already in the cause.*
> —Henri Louis Bergson

> *The definition of insanity is continuing to do the same thing over and over and then expecting different results.*
> —Most commonly attributed to Albert Einstein

When you build a house, it's very important that you start with a strong foundation. It is my belief that finding your way back to health starts with a strong foundation as well. In your case, you must begin armed with knowledge. Why did you get sick? Why do you have symptoms? If you don't understand the cause of your condition, how can you make different decisions for your health in the future? How can you avoid what brought you to where you are if you don't understand it?

To begin our journey toward understanding the body in a more holistic way, we have to start with the basics. There are two points of view of health and the human body: mechanistic and vitalistic.

MECHANISTIC VS. VITALISTIC APPROACHES TO SYMPTOM TREATING AND HEALING

The mechanistic view

This view, which dominates health care in the United States today, tends to ignore the *cause* of the illness or condition. Its focus is primarily symptom-based. Think of your body as a car. It is made up of parts. When your car won't start one morning, it is taken to the mechanic, where the part or parts most likely causing the specific problem are examined and replaced if necessary. The alternator may be broken, but the rest of the car still works. Therefore, the alternator is fixed or replaced. This is how mechanistic health care works. I hesitate to even call this model "health care." It is focused mainly on "disease care" and, more specifically, on emergency care.

What do I mean by this? In traditional health care today, the body is typically ignored—except for periodically being tested and examined for problems by your doctor—until a sign or symptom of malfunction rears its ugly head. At this point, you make an appointment to see your doctor and the symptom is examined, diagnosed, and managed. The focus of all treatments seems to be symptom-oriented: isolate the broken or malfunctioning body part or organ located by symptoms, fix it or numb it with surgery or medications, or remove the offending part(s). Even "preventative" care has more to do with early detection, rather than promoting health and vitality *before* problems arise.

The philosophy is a simple one: if there is pain, numb it. If the patient is not sleeping at night, force their body to sleep at night by drugging it. If the patient has pain all over, give them painkillers. If they appear to also suffer from, let's say, irritable bowel syndrome (IBS), the relationship between these two sets of symptoms is seldom examined and tend to be treated separately. The patient will be given a thorough exam and probably go through some tests, and in the end, a different doctor will most likely manage the IBS with different medications. We are bombarded with ads for designer medications for every condition under the sun. Have you heard these words lately? "Ask your doctor about..." The message is clear: manage every symptom. Squash it, numb it, interrupt it, silence it, or cut it out.

If the mechanistic way of doing things worked, it is obvious that the United States would be full of healthy people. We have some of the best hospitals, the best doctors, and more pharmaceutical companies than you can throw a rock at. A good example of this is the great American tradition of direct-to-consumer advertising, where drugs are marketed directly to the public. You know the ads. It typically goes like this: attractive actors (or sometimes even celebrities like Sally Field) ask you if you suffer from a list of symptoms. You do? Well, presto! They have the answer in the form of some drug. This is followed by members of the public being urged to "ask their doctor" about the drug by name, finally followed by a long list of side effects rambled off very rapidly, resembling a witch's book of spells. Drug companies like Pfizer spend around six billion dollars a year on this type of marketing.

Are Americans healthier because of this? Not exactly. A new report done in 2013 prepared by a panel of doctors, epidemiologists, and other researchers at the request of the National Research Council and the Institute of Medicine, found a "strikingly consistent and pervasive" pattern of poorer health of Americans at all stages of life. In fact, Americans' health ranked below that of sixteen other developed nations. We may live longer than we used to, but what is the quality of those extended lives?

The vitalistic view

The vitalistic viewpoint takes a very different approach. The body is seen as more than the sum of its parts. It is understood that the body is a masterful, intelligent system where every part affects every other part. It is studied in terms of its dynamic connections with its environment. It boils down to: fix the whole, including its environment, and the parts will take care of themselves.

When we study the body by looking at smaller and smaller parts, we may find certain organs or systems that are not working properly. For example, a patient may suffer from diabetes if the pancreas isn't producing insulin. However, the *cause* of the pancreas not producing insulin is rarely addressed. When a giant corporation finds itself in hot water for some reason, blame is usually not laid at the feet of each individual worker all the way down to the mailroom and cleaning staff. Rather, the top management of the company is scrutinized first, together with its policies. In much the same way, it makes more sense to examine a malfunctioning body from the top down. View the body as a corporation where the brain and spinal cord form the central nervous system (CNS); that is the CEO.

YOUR AMAZING BODY

I often ask patients whether they appreciate how incredibly intelligent their bodies are. This is often met with scorn and annoyance by those with less-than-stellar health. People who suffer from fibromyalgia often have a sense that their bodies have betrayed them in some way. They feel as if they can't trust their bodies, since those very bodies have let them down. It is a source of pain and it keeps them from doing the things they love, which is understandable. But let's step back for a moment and look at this differently. The body of a patient who suffers from fibromyalgia is under immense ongoing stress. It doesn't have the life-giving energy available to it that normal people's have. Each cell is functioning under stress. Yet it chugs on like the little engine that could. It is essential that you regain a sense of love and respect for this amazing living organism that allows you to live another day, as this is part of the recovery process.

Do you think your body isn't all it's cracked up to be? Let's look at the some of the things this body of yours can do. Your body was designed to survive (sometimes horrific) injuries even if a large part of your internal organs was removed. The human body may appear fragile, but it's possible to survive even with the removal of the stomach, the spleen, 75 percent of the liver, 80 percent of the intestines, one kidney, one lung, and virtually every organ from the pelvic and groin area. You might not feel too great, but the missing organs wouldn't kill you.

Your body is innately intelligent. It does many, many things at once. If I asked you to consciously and accurately monitor your blood pressure, heart rate, blood sugar levels, and temperature for ten minutes, it would be impossible to do so without the help of some serious technology. Yet your body does this and more every millisecond of every day and night without your having to give it any thought. We can think of the human body as an organized collection of infinitely intelligent cells. Each cell is like an elaborate biochemical computer. It has its own power-management and information-processing structures. It continuously communicates with its neighbors and the environment.

Each cell is an individual organism. Under certain conditions it may even be capable of living outside of the body. Most cells have a complete copy of the body's genetic information and are theoretically capable of recreating the whole human body. The magnitude of information-processing activity inside the human body is amazing. The cell reproduction processes require terabytes of genetic information to be copied every second within the body. And the protein formation and other functions in cells can be several orders of magnitude more information-intensive. The power consumption of a single cell corresponds to about 10^7 chemical reactions per second.[5]

The smartest scientist in the world cannot create life from scratch, or a hair from nothing. Your body serves you well. You may be thinking that while all this information is nifty, it does not explain why your body somehow became messed up and now has you feeling like dog poop every day. Nor does it explain why it's not repairing itself already. This is a valid point! As one of my patients once so eloquently put it: "awesome body my behind Dr. K!" I understood her frustration just like I understand yours. There has to be a reason *why* this supposedly amazing, self-healing and self-regulating body of yours has gone on the fritz. Let's look at why this happens.

WHACK THAT MOLE WITH OUR DESIGNER DRUG: THE PERILS OF SYMPTOM MANAGEMENT

Would you guess that our bodies were designed to be healthy? I have news for you. Your body, amazing though it may be, was *not* designed to be healthy. Your body was not designed to be sick either, of course. It was designed to *survive*. Symptoms, however unpleasant, were designed to alert your brain of problems that might ultimately threaten your survival. Think of pain as a fire alarm in a burning house. Have you ever woken up to that screeching, bone-chilling noise? The smart thing to do is to find out if the house is in fact on fire, call 911, put the fire out if possible, and if you can't, to get yourself and your loved ones out of the house and to safety. The firefighters will contain the fire and hopefully locate its source. The stupid thing to do would be to wet a towel and place it over the annoying fire alarm in order to stop the noise. Yet we treat symptoms as annoyances that must be managed.

This is a very dangerous game to play. Herbert A. Roberts, MD, put it this way: "The immediate effect of this method of treatment is a suppression but if persisted in and continued over a period of time it has the effect of driving the vital energy to express itself in some other form, and usually in a deeper and more vital organ."[6] Translated: if you suppress a symptom today, you will eventually have to pay the piper. Suppressed symptoms lead to bigger, more serious problems down the road. This never fails to happen.

You don't arrive at healing by addressing the symptom (unless the symptom is immediately trauma-related—for instance, a cut). To do so would be the equivalent of addressing the reaction instead of the initial action in order to prevent the reaction. Healing entails an understanding of the universal law of cause and effect, which states that every action has a reaction and every cause an effect. Suppression eventually will be expressed. Suppression always creates an outlet to express. When you suppress a thing, you will be forced to hold on to that thing. It's not seen at the surface, but it's there underneath, picking up steam or momentum with which to express itself when the time is ripe. Think of it as a volcano gathering strength below the surface of the earth, or a hurricane off the coast of Florida, growing more ominous and powerful by the day, even if the beaches still seem sunny and safe.

You may rightly ask what you are supposed to do if you are in pain, then. You have a life, job, family, and friends. Are you supposed to bite the bullet every day and just suffer? Live in pain? This is not what I am suggesting. To live each day with intolerable pain would be excruciating and unhealthy in itself. However, it is my hope that this book will give you information about your condition and how you got to the place where you are today, as this may translate to moving one step closer to living without the need for daily pain management. In my clinic, I never, ever tell patients to stop taking their medications. However, we work closely with their medical doctors so that when the patient feels ready, their pain medication is adjusted and eventually eliminated altogether when possible.

Now. Let's talk about why our bodies get overwhelmed and how we get sick.

THAT OVERUSED WORD: STRESS

> *I was a little excited but mostly blorft. 'Blorft' is an adjective I just made up that means 'Completely overwhelmed but proceeding as if everything is fine and reacting to the stress with the torpor of a possum.' I have been blorft every day for the past seven years.*
> —*Tina Fey*

My dad, who is one of my greatest mentors and has been a chiropractor for forty-one years, likes to tell his patients that their stress will end the day the lid on their coffin is closed. What he means by this is that stress is an unavoidable part of human existence. We can no more avoid stress than we can avoid breathing. However, once you understand that it is not stress *itself* that makes us sick, it may bring you some peace and comfort. Who wants to be a victim of stress? Wouldn't you rather be the one in control? The good news is that you *are* in control.

We usually think of stress as all bad, but that is not necessarily true. Let's look at what stress *actually* is. The official definition of stress in medicine is: "the result produced when a structure, system, or organism is acted upon by a stressor; when stress occurs in quantities that the system cannot handle, it produces pathological changes." In layperson's terms, stress technically is *any* change that requires your body to change in order to process it. If you follow this logic, even eating a banana can cause the body stress. If you didn't swallow it and it became stuck in your throat, it could suffocate you, resulting in your untimely demise. In addition, if your body could not digest and eliminate it, it would make you very sick. Although we typically associate stress with an emotional upset, there are actually three kinds of stress that affect your health: physical, chemical, and emotional stress.

PHYSICAL STRESS

Physical stress comes from the world outside of your body. A car accident is an excellent example of a physical stress that may contribute to a patient's developing fibromyalgia. In 1997, a team of investigators led by Israeli researcher Dan Buskila, MD, reported on a study of the relationship between cervical spine injuries and the onset of fibromyalgia and found that fibromyalgia was thirteen times more likely to occur following a neck injury than an injury to the lower extremities.[8]

Patients will often tell me that although they had a car accident, it was insignificant and could not have caused significant injuries to their necks because they (or the car that hit them) were driving really slowly when it happened and there was little damage to their vehicles. Sometimes they think it's not worth mentioning during their history since it happened a long time ago. Please note that *the force of the impact or the time that has gone by since the injury often has no effect on the extent of the injury.*

One researcher has shown that when a thirty-five-hundred–pound car traveling at ten miles an hour strikes the rear of another car, it may transmit to this car a force of twenty-five tons. The person in the car that is struck continues to move forward while their head, being hinged at the neck, snaps backward. The average head weighs about eight pounds, and the cervical vertebrae (the bones of the neck) are very delicate; the force pushing the head backward is even greater than you might believe since the base of the neck acts as a fulcrum and the leverage is applied near the top of the head.

Therefore, the head snaps back with the equivalent of several tons of force without any support, since the muscle control of the neck is caught off guard. The end result, with the neck in acute hyperextension, is that the nerve root (where the nerve exits the spinal cord) is caught in a pincer between the superior and inferior facets (the special posterior joints of the spine).[9] Car accidents are not the only culprits. The cervical spine may be injured in a number of different ways: falls, birth injuries, long-forgotten childhood injuries, sports injuries, or any injuries that caused you to suffer a concussion or cervical spine (neck) injury.

Another way patients may be injured is through general anesthesia. When the muscles that normally hold the bones of the neck in a safe position are paralyzed by the anesthesia, it is easy for the neck to be injured, especially if the neck is bent back in order for the breathing tube to be inserted in the patient's throat. Injuries to the neck are so prevalent in patients who suffer from fibromyalgia that we will devote more space to the neck and nervous system elsewhere in this book.

Other examples of physical injuries include injuries to the cranial nerves (the nerves that control your senses, like hearing, sight, and smell). I have a patient (let's call her Bonnie) who was doing very well after her third month of treatment. Her big goal after recovery was to go to Florida on a vacation with a girlfriend. After a trip to an amusement park where she went on some of the spinning rides, she suffered severe nausea and dizziness for a month after returning home. The cranial nerves dealing with her balance had been injured. Such injuries can also be caused by excessive visual or auditory stimulation. (Interestingly enough, she underwent several needless, grueling tests ordered by her MDs targeting her digestive system before she finally happened to mention to me one day that her nausea had started *immediately* following the ride at the amusement park.)

The body was designed to heal after injuries. However, sometimes the body is already under stress at the time of a physical injury, making it harder to recover afterward. Think how much easier it is for a string to snap if it is pulled very taut. For example, let's say that you are going through a divorce. One night you are particularly upset. You are driving home after an emotionally wrenching day that ended with a nasty phone call from your soon-to-be ex, and then to top it all off, you are hit from behind by another car. The fact that you were under emotional stress at the time of the accident, causing your body to be tense, will make it much more likely that you will be injured by that car accident and make it more difficult to recover.

During a traumatic event, the nervous system goes into survival mode (exciting or turning on the sympathetic nervous system) and sometimes has difficulty reverting back into its normal, relaxed mode again (controlled by the parasympathetic nervous system). If your nervous system is stuck in survival mode, stress hormones such as cortisol are constantly released, causing an increase in blood pressure and blood sugar, which can in turn reduce the immune system's ability to heal. Physical symptoms start to manifest when the body is in constant distress. If you add a physical injury on top of these conditions, the body now enters a danger zone where healing does not occur as easily as it should.

CHEMICAL STRESS

We are blessed with free choice. Every day, we get to choose the things we eat and drink. Your body responds to every single thing you put into it, whether you swallow it, inject it, rub it on your skin, or inhale it. After it enters our bodies, the part of us that gets to choose, however, is no longer in control. Now it is up to your body to process what you just put into it. Did it add to your health, or take away from it? Elsewhere in this book, we will devote an entire chapter to nutrition and supplements. For now, nutrition deserves to be briefly mentioned. Food will either enhance your health or take away from it.

Medications can add tremendous stress to the already stressed body of a fibromyalgia patient. It is very important for every fibromyalgia patient who is taking a lot of medications to support their liver and kidneys with detoxification and nutritional supplements.

Another bad habit that many people in chronic pain cling to is smoking. You'd have to live under a rock to not know that smoking is bad for you. It is especially detrimental to those who suffer from fibromyalgia because it decreases oxygen to the brain and increases neurological injury. Alcohol and nicotine add to your toxic chemical load. It should go without saying that these vices are especially detrimental to patients who already suffer from fibromyalgia. Please note that even secondhand smoke, or smoke clinging to the clothes of someone next to you, will affect your brain oxygen levels.

In my experience, it is much harder for a patient to recover from any condition, fibromyalgia included, if they refuse to give up smoking. In addition to putting a tremendous stress on the lungs and decreasing oxygen to the brain, smoking will add toxins like heavy metals to your system that will interfere with your healing. A good example of this is cadmium. Cadmium is an extremely toxic metal commonly found in cigarettes that is very easily absorbed by the lungs. Cadmium may cause osteoporosis, arthritis, kidney pain, and a host of other unpleasant symptoms.

When a smoker enters care, I am decidedly more apprehensive of their recovery than with normal patients, unless the patient is able to undergo the difficult process of quitting smoking. Adding to your toxic load will not help you to feel better or to live a longer, better life. However, we understand that daily pain will sometimes cause people to make poor choices in health. It is very difficult to stop a bad habit that is nevertheless comforting if you are in pain. Judging, we are not. However, you will show your body tremendous love and support if you can stop these bad habits. If necessary, get professional help. I have found that hypnosis is especially helpful in kicking toxic habits, as it addresses not only the physical but also the emotional and powerful subconscious addiction.

DIET SUGARS: JUST GO FOR THE
SUGAR IF YOU MUST

I wanted to address diet drinks and sugar separately. Most notably, I want to mention aspartame. Aspartame is the technical name for the brand names Spoonful, NutraSweet, Equal, and Equal-Measure. It was discovered by accident in the sixties when James Schlatter, a chemist, was testing an ulcer drug. Aspartame accounts for over 75 percent of the adverse reactions to food additives reported to the FDA. Many of these reactions are very serious, including seizures and death.

Aspartame is found in almost every single brand of gum, something that patients who suffer from fibromyalgia are particularly fond of in my experience. It is also found in diet sodas and drinks and in many other foods, including some children's vitamins. Recently, the EPA found aspartame to be a potentially dangerous chemical along with BPA (BisphenolA), which you've no doubt heard a lot about in the news lately. BPA is the harmful chemical that is often released by plastic cups, toys, and containers, especially when heated up. Most parents now know that their baby's bottle should be BPA-free. However, have you heard about aspartame being bad for you in mainstream media lately? Not so much.

WHAT IS ASPARTAME MADE OF?

Aspartame is made of three components: 50 percent phenylalanine, 40 percent aspartic acid, and 10 percent methanol (wood alcohol). In the body, methanol breaks down into formaldehyde (embalming fluid) and formic acid. While going through school and doing human dissection, formaldehyde was one of the smells that clung to me and my classmates in a stinky chemical fog that seemed to repel the public. After a while, it is almost impossible to remove the smell from your skin. It is used to preserve cadavers and acts as a preservative inside of the body. Today, our bodies are exposed to so many preservatives that they are actually taking much longer to decay after death. Gross, right? While it used to take a body about eight years to crumble into dust (hence "dust to dust"), it can now take forty years or longer! Maybe it's just me, but I find this fact particularly creepy.

ASPARTIC ACID (40 PERCENT OF ASPARTAME)

Dr. Russell L. Blaylock, a professor of neurosurgery at the Medical University of Mississippi, published a book thoroughly describing the damage caused by the ingestion of too much aspartic acid. He makes use of almost five hundred scientific references to show how excess free amino acids such as aspartic acid and glutamic acid do damage to the human body. Monosodium Glutamate (MSG) is the Sodium Salt of Glutamic Acid or Glutamate. Found in our food supply, it is causing serious chronic neurological disorders and a ton of other unwanted symptoms, such as numbness, vertigo, and seizures.

HOW ASPARTATE (AND GLUTAMATE) CAUSE DAMAGE

Aspartame releases aspartate during digestion. Aspartate and glutamate (MSG is the sodium salt of glutamate) act as neurotransmitters (think of them as chemical taxis) in the brain by facilitating the transmission of information from neuron to neuron. Too much aspartate or glutamate in the brain kills certain neurons by allowing the influx of too much calcium into the cells. This influx triggers excessive amounts of free radicals, which kill the cells. The neural cell damage that can be caused by excessive aspartate and glutamate is why they are referred to as "excitotoxins." They "excite" or stimulate the neural cells to death. My colleagues and I have observed that few things will injure the nervous system as rapidly and completely as aspartame.

Splenda is another culprit. It is marketed in such a savvy way that you would swear it's made by Mother Nature herself. It is often included in products labeled as "all-natural." However, Splenda is chlorinated sugar and is anything but natural. There have been no long-term human studies on the safety of Splenda; however, several issues have been raised about Splenda. According to a study from Duke University, Splenda "suppresses beneficial bacteria and directly affects the expression of the transporter isozymes that are known to interfere with the bioavailability of drugs and nutrients. Furthermore, these effects occur at Splenda doses that contain sucralose levels that are approved by the FDA for use in the food supply."[10]

A great natural alternative is the sweetener stevia, which is derived from a plant. Stevia was first discovered in 1500 and widely used for hundreds of years by American Indians. In the early '70s, as problems with other sweeteners emerged, Japan started widely using stevia. Today, it accounts for 40 percent of all sweetened products produced in Japan. Numerous studies in the United States and Europe found stevia to be safe and even beneficial. Your local health-food store should carry this sweetener in its natural form (I recommend the KAL brand). If you chew on a stevia plant leaf, you will find that it is naturally sweet. A great rule of thumb is that the more humans interfere with food, the worse it is for you.

COSMETICS

A large number of personal care and cosmetic products, including deodorants, lotions, makeup, and even baby shampoos, contain chemicals that are linked to cancer, learning disabilities, birth defects, asthma, and other health problems. The average woman today uses about a dozen personal care products daily, containing more than one hundred and twenty chemicals. I like to tell my patients that if you can't eat it, you should not put it on your skin. We forget that the skin is not an impenetrable covering surrounding our bodies, but a living, breathing organ rich with blood supply that serves as a portal of entry straight into the body.

If you suffer from fibromyalgia, I suggest you take extra care to protect your body from toxic chemicals such as lead (still contained in many lipsticks), phthalates (industrial chemicals contained in almost every cosmetic and personal care product and that have been shown to disrupt the endocrine system), sulfates, heavy metals, and countless other harmful chemicals. A great resource that I recommend to my patients is the Environmental Working group's "skin deep" website (http://www.ewg.org/skindeep).

EWG's Skin Deep database gives you practical solutions to protect yourself and your family from everyday exposure to chemicals. It was launched in 2004 to create online safety profiles for cosmetics and personal care products. Their aim is to fill in where industry and government leave off. Using this website, you can look up the safety and ingredients of most of the products that you use, and the effects the chemicals contained in these products have on the human body.

That being said, I don't recommend that you obsess about the thousands of chemicals you *can't* avoid. Even babies in utero have been shown to be exposed to harmful chemicals. It is impossible to completely avoid our toxic environment. However, educate yourself on the products that you use daily and make better choices where you can. For example, instead of buying only organic produce, look up the "dirtiest" fruits and vegetables (see chapter 11 for a complete list), and try to buy these only if they are certified organically grown.

It is a good rule of thumb to detoxify the whole body at least quarterly. This can be done in many ways. I like the Isagenix nine-day detoxification, and a *good quality* ionic footbath (not all are created equal). I also like doing this through eating a very pure diet, as described in chapter 11.

EMOTIONAL STRESS

Although we often blame emotional stress on the actions of people around us as well as the ups and downs of life in general, it is actually the one stress completely in our power to control. Emotional stress is nothing more than feelings that don't feel good, originating from our thoughts. Every person has a unique filter through which they experience the world. Whether we experience something as pleasant or unpleasant, good or bad, happy or sad has much to do with our upbringing, our ethical values, and that which we hold dear. I had a mentor who used to tell his patients something I will never forget: "You can spit in my face, but you cannot *make* me mad." We can't control the actions of others. However, we can control the *feelings* their actions cause us to feel.

Close your eyes and "feel" your thoughts for a second. Every thought, if we focus on our bodies, tends to be accompanied by an actual physical sensation; these sensations are generally distinctly pleasant or unpleasant. Close your eyes and focus on a thought. Now pay attention to the physical sensation that thought generates in your body. Is there a nice warm feeling in your chest, about where you imagine your heart is located, or do you have an unpleasant feeling in the pit in your stomach? Does it feel like your heart is being squeezed with fear and dread or that a heavy weight is resting on your chest? Are you feeling boredom, annoyance, terror, or frustration?

EMOTIONAL STRESS AND HOW IT AFFECTS YOUR NERVOUS SYSTEM

Let's imagine that your brain is a computer. You have hardware (brain cells, nerves, white matter, gray matter, the spinal cord, and so on), and software (the signals you can't *see*, but that you know are there). If you decide to pick up a glass of water, your nerves respond to the decision made by the great CEO, the brain. They pass the command down to the muscles of your arm and fingers. These muscles and tendons contract and relax to move the bones, and, presto! You are holding a glass.

You have a conscious mind and a subconscious mind. The conscious mind resides in the cerebral cortex, which is a thin layer of nerve cells about one eighth of an inch thick that surrounds your brain. The conscious mind is your thinking, judging, and decision-making mind. This is the area we use when we make choices. This area is fed by the five senses (what you see, hear, smell, taste, and feel) and by information entering your mind through the cranial nerves discussed elsewhere in this book. When you learn to ride a bike, that information is programmed in the cerebral cortex where you can access it at any time.

Over time, as your body builds muscle memory and the actions of riding a bike or walking become routine, the knowledge is dumped in the area underneath this layer, the cerebrum. Occasionally, these bits of information may not be easily accessible (for example, when you forget someone's name). For the most part, however, the information in the conscious mind is readily available. Think of it as the thinking mind, or a vast library of information. When you are born, the conscious mind is a blank slate. As we have our first human experiences as babies, this area is programmed. We may learn that the appearance of our mother's face is shortly followed by comfort and food, and that if we cry, our demands are met. We may also learn useful bits of information. For example: if we touch a hot curling iron or a pan this brings pain, and it should be avoided for the rest of our life.

The subconscious mind is the area that runs our bodies, driven by one singular, razor-sharp goal: survival. It is the lower "animal" part of our brain at the base of our skull. When we are born, this area is already filled with all we need built in for survival. The newborn baby does not need to be taught how to regulate his or her insulin, how to digest milk, or how to breathe. This part cannot think, judge, or

reason. It simply responds to what is being programmed into the conscious mind.

Imagine that you are driving along one day and notice a police car
with flashing lights in your rear-view mirror. You may become scared.
Your subconscious or automatic nervous system will respond by
going into survival mode. Your heart rate will go up, your hands may
sweat on the steering wheel, and your stomach may pull into a knot.
When the police car passes you, you will take a deep breath and laugh
about how silly you were. The body usually will take a few minutes to
respond, but eventually your heart will slow down, and you may even
feel relaxed enough to stop and grab something to eat.

The subconscious mind cannot distinguish between a real threat
to your survival and a fake one. It cannot distinguish between the
present and the past. Think of a deep emotional wound as a virus
in your computer. Even though you visited the website where your
computer was infected months ago, the virus will continue to do
its annoying thing as if it had been infected today. When your computer was infected does not matter. When very traumatic things
happen to us, it is as if we play a CD with a scratch on it over and
over. The subconscious mind responds to this traumatic event as a
threat to its survival. Remember, to your subconscious mind, the
traumatic event and the feelings it caused may as well be a real-life
threat, like an angry bear. It is responding perfectly to *inappropriate information*.

Let's pretend for a minute that when you were ten years old,
your abusive alcoholic father hit your mother. Unfortunately, you witnessed this event. Your subconscious mind responded to the intense
fear the situation created as if your life were being threatened. It is
still responding to this memory with the typical tools of survival. You
are scared, your blood pressure is elevated, you can't eat, your muscles are tense and ready to fight. Only...there is no abusive father,
simply the *memory* of him, churning destructively and unnoticed in
the subconscious mind.

Your subconscious mind is responding to this memory as if it is a present danger. It cannot distinguish between present and past. Like the virus in your computer, it is ever-present, all the time, as if on a loop. To your subconscious mind, this is still happening *right now*. It is causing your digestive system to shut down with your stomach in knots, your heart to pound with anxiety, and your blood pressure to be elevated.

Since you are not consciously *aware* of this memory very much alive in the subconscious, wreaking havoc upon your body, these symptoms make no sense. They seem out of place and will usually eventually cause you to seek medical help. If you were to tell your doctor that you are scared and anxious all the time, you can't sleep, and your stomach hurts when you eat, he or she would most probably prescribe anti-anxiety medications, sleeping medications, or antidepressants and refer you to a specialist for your digestive problems.

You are now chemically masking your physiological response to this buried memory. See the problem with this approach? The automatic (or autonomic) nervous system is so important that we will devote an entire chapter to it elsewhere. However, just know that there are upper cervical (neck) injuries that may cause your body to respond with the same fight-or-flight response, stuck in an endless loop.

One study found that 20 percent of all people suffering from fibromyalgia also suffered from post-traumatic stress disorder (PTSD).[11] Once called shell shock, PTSD is a serious condition that can develop after a person has experienced or witnessed a traumatic or terrifying event in which serious physical harm occurred or was threatened. PTSD is a lasting result of a traumatic experience that caused intense fear, helplessness, or horror, such as a sexual or physical assault, the unexpected death of a loved one, or an accident, war, or natural disaster. Patients who suffered sexual or physical abuse suffer from a high burden of stress upon their nervous systems and bodies, and are much more likely to develop chronic conditions such as fibromyalgia.

Most people who experience a traumatic event will have reactions that may include shock, anger, nervousness, fear, and even guilt. These reactions are common, and for most people they go away over time. However, for a person with PTSD, these feelings continue and may even increase, becoming so strong that they keep the person from living a normal, happy life. People with PTSD have symptoms for longer than one month and cannot function as well as they did before the event occurred.

SO HOW DOES ONE AVOID...LIFE?

When I explain the effect emotional stress may have on their bodies to my patients, I almost always get this question: How does one avoid the bad things in life that seem to happen to all of us sooner or later? Remember, it is not *what* happens to us that makes us physically sick; it is our *feelings* about these things that get our bodies stuck. So, are you supposed to stop feeling then? Just flip that handy-dandy "emotions off" switch in the back of your head? We are all human, after all. Although your emotions are 100 percent under your control, it is difficult to leave behind a lifetime of programming. When someone dies, we miss them. It makes us sad. When another driver is rude to us on the road, we get angry. How do we change the way we naturally respond to stress...with feeling? How do you friggin' neutralize negative feelings?

STEP 1: MAKE THE LINK

Understanding that feelings can make you physically sick is the first step. The founder of chiropractic, Dr. D.D. Palmer, used to say, "Be very careful who you rent the upstairs to." When you learn to watch your thoughts, based on the feelings you are feeling, you can begin to correct them. Awareness is the first step to healthier thinking. Most people just feel what they feel with abandon, with little thought of the consequence that those intense emotions may have upon their health. Every feeling has an effect upon your body; it can be a good effect or a bad effect.

STEP 2: QUIT ACTING LIKE A HONEY BADGER

If you are unfamiliar with the famous "honey badger" video on YouTube, please go watch it now. If you can't, I will sum it up for you here but will scarcely do it justice. "Honey Badger" is a famous short YouTube video taking a look at the tough honey badger from Africa, narrated by a hilarious guy called Randall. The narrator talks about how tough and fearless the honey badger is. For example, it is shown killing and eating a poisonous snake while the narrator constantly remarks that the strong little "honey badger don't care." Honey badger may be too tough to care, but you aren't.

You have to acknowledge your feelings. As children, we are often taught that big boys and girls don't cry. It is implied that it is better to "suck it up," to keep our chins up, and to get over it. However, when you suppress an emotion, it will be expressed as a physical symptom. It will implode. Think of expressing your emotions as a pressure valve. It will keep your feelings from becoming toxic.

I am not necessarily advocating that you confront people to their face; although this may be appropriate in some cases, it may also cause you too much anxiety. I, for one, despise confrontation. It reminds me of a funny joke here in the South: "I don't talk badly about people to their face. No, ma'am. My mamma raised me right. I do it *behind* their backs." I would rather drive needles through my skin with a hammer than confront people face to face. If you are like me and you would rather stuff your emotions down, I feel your pain. However, this is not a healthy way to live.

You have to learn to at least *own* your feelings. "When you said X to me, it made me feel Y. I understand that you did not necessarily mean to make me feel Y. These are just my feelings, which I am owning and taking responsibility for." Another great way of expressing your feelings is merely saying them out loud, even if no one else is around to hear you. I like to do this while I am driving or in the shower; that cuts down on the chances of other people thinking I have lost my marbles because I'm talking to myself. The mere act of saying something out loud counts as healthy expression. Think of it being said out loud with emotion as a release of negative energy from your body. Another solution is to write a letter or e-mail, even if you never send it. Many people find journaling helpful.

STEP 3: NEUTRALIZE THE ACID

Think back to your chemistry class in high school. How do you neutralize an acidic solution? You simply add an alkaline substance or solution. Think of your negative feelings as acid. It is corrosive and will eat away at you and your health unless neutralized. Whenever you find your thoughts about a memory to cause a negative emotion, mentally examine it until you can find some good in what happened.

Sometimes the only good you can find is the lesson you learned from that experience. Your lesson may be to not repeat that mistake, or to learn from the unpleasant feeling and vow to do better in the future, or maybe not to do unto others as has been done to you. Find at least one good thing in every unpleasant experience. It has to be there, by the law of polarity. Bad cannot exist without some good. The silver lining is there; just look for it.

My dad once had a patient whose husband was killed in front of her during a robbery. She asked him what good there was in that. His answer? *She* was not killed. That may seem like a small thing, but it was a significant blessing amid that tragedy. While this is an extreme example, you get my drift. Find the nugget of good and acknowledge it. Of course, it is best to do this right away. Try not to spend months or years working through negative things that could be handled immediately. Even if it feels like you are just going through the motions, it is still incredibly effective. A little bit of positivity goes a very long way.

STEP 4: SELFISHLY FORGIVE OTHERS

Forgiveness is the fragrance that the violet sheds on the heel that has crushed it.
—*Mark Twain*

The weak can never forgive. Forgiveness is the attribute of the strong.
—*Gandhi*

Forgiveness is a gift you give yourself.
—*Suzanne Summers*

When you forgive, you in no way change the past—but you sure do change the future.
—*Bernard Meltzer*

The last step is forgiveness. People sometimes resist this step, since it feels as if they are condoning what was done to them by forgiving it. "It was not OK. I will not imply it was OK by forgiving them." Choose to look at it differently, however. Forgiveness is actually a very empowering action that will speed up your healing. It does not imply that you condone what was done to you. It simply means that you are choosing to let go. It is a very peaceful action, bringing you great return upon the investment of energy it takes to forgive. After all, what are you really letting go of? Anger. Grief. Resentment. Why would you choose to hang on to these negative emotions? Hatred is an acid that destroys its own container. Picture your hands opening and letting go of broken glass you were tightly holding on to, causing you pain. Just let go. Let it fall to the ground.

Forgiveness must be heartfelt, and more than just words spoken. While it takes a strong person to say "sorry," it takes an even stronger person to forgive. Forgiveness can be instant, or a gentle, slow eroding of negative emotions as you keep focusing on any positives that came from the experience. Forgive the person, not the act. You will be healthier for it. You will be freer. Cut the ties that bind you with the most powerful sword in the world: forgiveness. Nothing binds you to a fellow human being more snugly than hatred.

STEP 5: FORGIVE YOURSELF

I have learned that the person I have to ask
for forgiveness from the most is myself.
You must love yourself.
You have to forgive yourself, every day, whenever
you remember a shortcoming, a flaw, you
have to tell yourself, 'That's just fine.'
You have to forgive yourself so much, until you don't even
see those things anymore. Because that's what love is like.
—C. Joy Bell

I have noticed that my patients are hardest on themselves. We sometimes find it much easier to forgive others than ourselves. We somehow feel that if only we can beat ourselves up hard enough, we can go back in time and undo our bad decisions. Not marry that jerk. Not say hurtful things. Not take that dead-end job. Finish school. Never start smoking. Not have our hearts broken by people who should never have had the power to do so in the first place. Our lists of regrets are usually long and tough to admit. Yet we never let ourselves forget our own mistakes.

Please understand, we can only forgive others to the extent to which we can forgive ourselves. Do you understand how profound this is? The harder we are on ourselves, the harder we are on those around us, those we love. Be extra kind to yourself. Imagine yourself to be a student, moving through life's various classes. Sometimes we fail. Sometimes we fall down. A mistake is only a lesson waiting to be learned. Be as kind to you as you are to your most beloved friend or pet. Messing up is part of being human.

THE NERVOUS SYSTEM: THE BUBBLE WRAP THAT PROTECTS AGAINST LIFE'S HARD KNOCKS

The most effective way to protect your body against physical, chemical, and emotional stress is to make sure that your nervous system is healthy. Your nervous system is the system that absorbs all the shocks of life. If this system is overwhelmed, stressed, and maxed out, the body will get injured pretty easily. When we rehabilitate a patient's nervous system, it is very easy for him or her to re-injure it in the beginning. Even getting up from the treatment table may re-injure it. We do not mean "injure" as in, for example, falling down. "Injuries" include *any* change to the nervous system. For example: in order to even sit up after lying down, your blood pressure has to rise. If your nervous system is unhealthy, this can be too taxing for it, and it can be "injured". Typically, the nervous system of a patient who suffers from fibromyalgia is especially fragile.

Acupuncture, chiropractic (gentle chiropractic techniques, in your case), light exercise if your body permits it, a healthy whole-food diet with plenty of fruits, vegetables, and healthy oils, and supplementation (such as magnesium) are all things that will strengthen your nervous system. (Please read chapter 9 on supplementation.)

Of course, if you are very sick, it is not possible to start exercising, nor is it advised. If you suffer from fibromyalgia, you must learn to listen to your body. Do *not* exercise through pain any more than you would run a marathon with a broken leg. Start very, very slow with any exercise and work your way up if you are tolerating it well. Swimming, walking and slow yoga are good examples of exercise you can possibly tolerate.

CHAPTER 5

YOUR CERVICAL SPINE: UNDERSTANDING THE MOST COMMON CAUSE OF FIBROMYALGIA

> *For thousands of years professions that ministered to the sick disregarded the centrifugal or inside force (Innate Intelligence) and searched the heavens and the earth in a vain attempt to externally find the cause of disease.*
> —B. J. Palmer
>
> *Every organ in your body is connected to the one under your hat.*
> —B. J. Palmer

Some physicians (including myself) believe that there are different types of fibromyalgia. Some think that there is only one main form of fibromyalgia, also known as primary fibromyalgia, which is responsible for the wide variety of symptoms in FMS patients. It is my opinion that regardless of some of the other contributing factors, the cervical spine (neck) and autonomic (automatic) nervous system are almost always involved in fibromyalgia. Sometimes it is the sole cause, and sometimes it is part of what my colleague and friend Dr. DeMartino (DCQN) refers to as "the perfect storm." It is a group of circumstances that came together and caused the collection of symptoms known as fibromyalgia to develop. I invite you to read this chapter and then to decide for yourself.

It is very important, when trying to understand how the human body works, to realize and appreciate how integral the central nervous system is to the body. When an embryo develops, the nervous system is the first tissue to differentiate or form. It is the system that runs the entire body. It controls every single function or task that your body performs. The brain is the captain; the spinal cord is the highway that carries the signals and commands to every cell and delivers feedback to this captain. It is the master control system. Every feeling of discomfort or pain involves the nervous system. In order for you to be healthy, this system has to be healthy.

Fibromyalgia is a global failure of the central nervous system. Almost every fibromyalgia patient who starts care in my clinic tells me that their body is "different" from other people's. They tend to process pain differently. Doctors seem to think that their symptoms present a challenge when trying to diagnose them. Often they are sensitive to medications and allergic to certain foods. They tend to be very reactive to stress of any kind. It is almost as if the body becomes uncooperative, hypersensitive, and unpredictable. It is puzzling and frustrating to health care practitioners and patients alike. However, although fibromyalgia is a complicated condition, there do seem to be common symptoms and a certain history that most patients with fibromyalgia share. One of the most common is a history of neck pain or trauma. Let's take a closer look at the cervical spine and its role.

CERVICAL SPINE TRAUMA AND FIBROMYALGIA

As mentioned before, people who suffer from cervical (neck) injuries are 13.3 times more likely to develop fibromyalgia than others.[12] While no exact percentages are known, it is my experience that the vast majority of patients who suffer from fibromyalgia also suffered from upper cervical trauma at some point. I would venture to put this number as high as 80 percent. For this reason, we are going to focus heavily on the involvement of this part of the spine in fibromyalgia.

It is important to note that the age of the injury is inconsequential. The mechanism of injury is often a car accident, but it can be attributed to many other mechanisms of injury, such as falls, birth trauma, or injury while under anesthesia (described in the "Physical Stress" section in the previous chapter). It is very important that you carefully examine your history from birth to adulthood when trying to understand what type of fibromyalgia you suffer from. Since the genetic cause of fibromyalgia is such a popular one, I want to introduce a possible link between the shape of the spinal cord, which may be genetic, and the predisposition for spinal injury following an accident.

CERVICAL SPINE STENOSIS: DOES IT MAKE YOU VULNERABLE TO DAMAGE?

Spinal stenosis (stenosis is the narrowing of a passage in the body) is a narrowing of the open canal that surrounds the spinal cord, or the foramina (bony opening) where the nerves exit the spine. This can put pressure on your spinal cord and the nerves that travel through the spine. Spinal stenosis occurs most often in the neck and lower back. While some people have no signs or symptoms, spinal stenosis can cause pain, tingling, muscle weakness, numbness, and problems with bladder or bowel function.

One study found that almost 50 percent of patients who suffered from fibromyalgia also suffered from cervical spine stenosis.[12] It has been shown through research that spinal cord stenosis predisposes patients to spinal cord injury. One study compared forty-two patients with confirmed spinal cord injuries to a hundred controls (people with no spinal cord injuries). They found that the healthy control group had *significantly* larger spinal canals (the space that contains and protects the spinal cord) than the patients with spinal cord injuries.[13] Another study puts the number of fibromyalgia patients with cord compression as high as 65 percent.[14]

It is postulated that two popular medications often prescribed for fibromyalgia, Lyrica and Cymbalta, actually address the symptoms of spinal cord pain rather than the indirect symptoms of fibromyalgia. The EU (European Union) approved Lyrica for central spinal cord pain. Of course, these medications simply address the *symptoms* of central spinal cord pain, and not the anatomical problem.

There are two types of cervical stenosis: congenital and degenerative.

CONGENITAL STENOSIS OF THE CERVICAL SPINAL CANAL

Some people are born with spinal stenosis. This is called *congenital stenosis*. They may not display any symptoms at a young age, but having a narrow canal to begin with places them at risk for pain and injuries later in life. Even a seemingly minor neck injury can set them up to have pressure against the spinal cord. People born with a narrow spinal canal often develop problems later in life because the canal tends to become narrower due to aging; and the resulting changes in the spine. These changes often involve the formation of *bone spurs* (small bony growths caused by abnormal pressure in the spine) that put pressure on the spinal cord.

DEGENERATIVE STENOSIS OF THE CERVICAL SPINAL CANAL

Degeneration is the most common cause of spinal stenosis. Wear and tear on the spine from aging and from repeated stress and strain may cause many problems in the cervical spine. The intervertebral discs can begin to collapse, shrinking the space between vertebrae. Because of this collapse, bone spurs may form and protrude into the spinal canal, reducing the space available to the spinal cord.

Another common degenerative cause of stenosis is calcification of the posterior longitudinal ligament of the cervical spine. The posterior longitudinal ligament is situated within the vertebral canal. It extends along the posterior surfaces of the bodies of the vertebrae, or building blocks that form the spine, and goes down all the way to the sacrum, or the very lowest part of the spine.

All of these conditions may cause narrowing of the canal, leading to neurological symptoms and making you more vulnerable to spinal cord damage.

GENETICS AND TRAUMA LINKED FOR THE FIRST TIME?

Until now, the obvious genetic propensity for fibromyalgia never fit together well with the evidence that cervical trauma causes fibromyalgia. Yet I noticed that patients suffering from fibromyalgia often shared two interesting things when they told me their health histories: although they often had a family member who suffered from fibromyalgia, it was not *triggered* until they suffered from some kind of trauma to the neck. This is of course not true for everybody, but quite commonly I find it to be the case. Congenital stenosis actually explains why both of these key factors are often present:

1. Cervical stenosis makes the patient much more vulnerable to any trauma, especially hyperextension (forcefully bending back) type trauma of the neck, as seen in whiplash injuries.

2. Females are more likely to develop foraminal (the opening through which nerves exit the spinal canal) stenosis than males. One study found that the diameters of these foramens were smaller in females at every level of the cervical spine.[15] This explains why so many more females than males suffer from fibromyalgia.

3. While it used to be believed that spinal stenosis was not genetic, it has been proven by several studies that such a genetic link does, in fact, exist. One study found twenty-four family members in one family who suffered from stenosis of the neck.[16] Another study found a genetic link in the case of calcification of the posterior longitudinal ligament of the spine (PLL), [17] a common cause of stenosis of the neck. Yet another study found a genetic link between common degenerative processes in the spine, such as stenosis.[18]

The above may all seem a bit complicated, but it is easy to sum up the important parts: Stenosis makes you vulnerable to an injury that very often will cause fibromyalgia. Females are more likely to suffer from stenosis, and it appears to often be genetic. This explains why females suffer from fibromyalgia more often than males, and why trauma to the neck, as well as genetics, may predispose you to suffer from fibromyalgia.

HOW DO I KNOW IF MY NECK IS THE PROBLEM?

Recognizing neck or upper-back trauma in a fibromyalgia patient can be tricky, since the majority of them either do not connect a past injury with their current diagnosis, or think that the injury was too insignificant to matter. Sometimes they may attribute it solely to the emotional stress that often accompanies a traumatic physical event, when both are actually to blame. I have seen this to be true especially in the case of domestic violence, where the emotional stress does play a role, but the physical injuries are dismissed as long healed. There are a few clues that tend to point to spinal trauma as a culprit:

- A known past injury (or injuries) to the neck and/or upper back

- Disc problems in the cervical spine, as seen on X-ray or MRI

- Pain that does not respond well to medications or other treatments, such as massage therapy, physical therapy, surgery, trigger point injections, or exercise

- Most will describe their extremities (hands and feet) as cold, aching, burning, or feeling as if they are "walking on glass"

- Severe headaches and/or migraines

- The pain will start out more locally but will eventually affect the entire spine, especially low back, and eventually the whole body

- Digestive problems

- "Foggy" feelings and feelings of confusion. Vision, hearing, speech, smell, balance, or taste may be affected

- Pain in shoulders and upper back

- Pain in the jaw/TMJ

- Central pain

CENTRAL PAIN

What is central pain? WebMD defines it thus: "Central pain syndrome is characterized by a mixture of pain sensations, the most prominent being a constant burning. The steady burning sensation is sometimes increased by light touch. Pain also increases in the presence of temperature changes, most often cold temperatures. A loss of sensation can occur in affected areas, most prominently on distant parts of the body, such as the hands and feet. There may be brief, intolerable bursts of sharp pain on occasion."

This pain is sharp, stabbing, tingling, shooting, or aching, and affected by temperature changes.

WEATHER CHANGES

Why does your body respond violently to changes in the weather? When patients suffer from central pain syndrome (CPS), their nervous systems actually change on several levels. In CPS, nociceptors (tiny pain receptors) and peripheral nerves become hypersensitive. Pain amplification in the spinal cord tends to increase, and the spinal cord's ability to filter pain decreases. These changes become evident when the patient's sensory nervous system is exposed to any change, such as cold, heat, or a drop in barometric pressure, which occurs when rain is coming in or the wind is blowing. This causes the sensory nervous system to respond to that change. Tissues will also swell as a result, making the patient's agony even worse.

HOW CAN I BE TESTED?

Please remember that while several tests may show problems in the neck, most doctors are not aware of the link between spinal problems and fibromyalgia. If you want to get clear answers about the health of your spine, you should probably not do so in the hope that it will affect your medical doctor's diagnosis or treatment of your fibromy-algia. We do think it is very valuable information, especially on your road to understanding your condition and in searching for treatments that will work, and in finding eventual relief. Here are some of the tests that may uncover cervical spine trauma fibromyalgia:

CERVICAL X-RAYS

Although X-rays can be useful to show overall damage and misalign-ment of the bones and other structures of the neck, it is important to have a *trained eye* look at those X-rays. Typically, misalignments of the bones (such as the bone shifting abnormally to the front or the back, or twisting out of position) and loss of the C-shaped curve (or lordotic curve) of the neck are seen as "normal degeneration" of the spine by most allopathic doctors. Health care professionals in the medical world are trained typically to not red-flag things that they often see and consider commonplace. Therefore, since degeneration is seen so often, it may be dismissed or only mentioned in passing.

A chiropractor is an example of a health care professional who has been trained with the philosophy that the integrity and overall health of the spine are crucial to the overall health of the person, and who will look for clues that other radiologists or doctors may dismiss. It is not a question of competency, but rather training and overall philosophies about health in general.

The clues to be looked for may include decreased disc space, misalignment of the spine, and degeneration of the spine, which is abnormal bone growth that the body uses to stabilize weakened areas, like casting a broken bone. These bones may also fuse together, or you could have a decreased curve of the neck called a hypolordotic curve, which appears as a straight neck or one curved in the wrong direction (think of forcefully straightening a banana). Lastly, you may have a misalignment of the upper first two bones in the neck, called the atlas and axis, or a misalignment of any of the bones in the neck.

In chiropractic, this is referred to as "subluxation." The word "subluxation" is derived from the Latin word "lux," or light, where "sub lux" means less than light, or less than perfect. Chiropractors, often viewed by the public as "bone poppers," actually do so much more than that. They believe that the health of the spine is vital, given the importance of the central nervous system to the health of the overall individual.

The drawback of X-rays is that they are not good at showing the soft tissues—nerves, discs, and ligaments—and will not show the health or integrity of the disc clearly. Also, make sure that these x-rays are taken while you are standing, since lying down will change the weight bearing of the spine and may hide injuries.

MRI

Magnetic resonance imaging allows health care professionals to take a look inside your body at the soft tissue structures of the spine, such as the discs. According to Carolyn R. McMakin (MA, DC), a doctor who specializes in the treatment of the neurological symptoms of this type of fibromyalgia, MRI studies of patients whose symptoms stem from spinal trauma will often show disc bulges (imagine a water balloon being squashed between two bricks). These disc bulges will most commonly appear between the fifth and sixth cervical bones or the sixth and seventh cervical bones, and less often between the fourth and fifth cervical bones.

Again, be aware that the average radiologist or doctor will see these changes as part and parcel of the "normal" aging process. Most MRIs are taken while the patient is lying down, which removes some of the normal weight that your discs carry when you are in an upright position. Although it is hard to find an imaging center that performs it, it is possible to do standing MRIs in the flexion (bending the neck forward) and extension (bending the neck back) positions, which will often show disc bulges that are "hiding" on conventional views.

FUNCTIONAL MRI

Functional magnetic resonance imaging or functional MRI (fMRI) is an MRI procedure that measures brain activity by detecting associated changes in blood flow. fMRI is used more in the research world than the clinical world. Although this technology is still in its infancy and not widely used yet, we did feel that it deserved a mention. Several groundbreaking studies using fMRI technology have shown that the brain of a patient suffering from fibromyalgia responds differently than the brains of healthy individuals. This makes them abnormally sensitive to pain. The next time someone tells you that fibromyalgia is "all in your head," you can first agree with them and then suggest that they Google these studies.

MYELOGRAM

A myelogram is an image that involves injecting contrast material by needle into the space around the spinal cord and nerve roots (the subarachnoid space) and then taking an image of it using a real-time form of X-ray called fluoroscopy. With the contrast material injected into this space, the radiologist is able to view and evaluate a very detailed picture of the status of the spinal cord, the nerve roots, and the meninges, the three membranes that cover the brain, spinal cord, and nerve roots.

The radiologist views the movement of contrast material in real time within the subarachnoid space as it is flowing and also takes X-rays of the contrast material around the spinal cord and nerve roots in order to show abnormalities in the spine. Although this type of imaging is very useful, injury to the soft tissues is always possible when a needle is used around the spine. For this reason, doctors prefer to order MRIs to view the spine.

PHYSICAL AND NEUROLOGICAL EXAM

According to Dr. McMakin, the developer of the frequency-specific microcurrent (FSM) treatment for the neurological symptoms of fibromyalgia, one of the important technologies I use in practice (more about our treatments in chapter 13), the patient suffering from cervical trauma fibromyalgia will have a significantly stronger patellar reflex (knee jerk reflex). Fibromyalgia that is not due to spinal trauma will have normal or even weaker reflexes than normal. In addition, she notes that cervical compression (pushing down on the top of the head) will cause pain in the neck and shoulders.

The fibromyalgia patient will usually show abnormalities of the cranial nerves IX (the glossopharyngeal nerve) and X (the vagus nerve). This may result in difficulty swallowing, a nasal sound to one's speech, coughing, and loss of sour and bitter tastes. The patient may also suffer from diplopia (seeing one object as two objects, most often with one eye covered), hypersensitivity of the upper chest and lateral upper arms, poor balance and/or coordination, tingling in the arms and legs, and weakness of the arm and leg muscles. Please remember that your doctor taking a careful history is vitally important when diagnosing fibromyalgia. Make sure he or she understands and note any past accidents, falls, neck problems, or head trauma.

Cervical trauma is sometimes not the only contributor to fibromyalgia, but may be only one of the factors leading to "the perfect storm" we referred to earlier. In the next chapter we will look at other possible contributors to fibromyalgia.

NEUROLOGICAL RELIEF CENTER TECHNIQUE AND TEST

This technique was developed by a chiropractor (Dr. Paul Whitcomb) in California. If you Google his name you will find that lots of controversy surrounds this doctor. I would like to take a brief moment to mention and explain this work, since it is, in my opinion, one of the easiest and most affordable ways to diagnose cervical trauma fibromyalgia.

Dr. Whitcomb became interested in fibromyalgia after he himself suffered from this condition for a long time. Through much research and different treatments, such as chiropractic, he eventually got better, but never forgot how much he suffered while sick. Some time after this, he had two patients start care in his office, both of whom developed fibromyalgia after being involved in the same car accident. Dr. Whitcomb figured that this was too great a coincidence and set out to examine their upper cervical spines, where he noticed similar injuries. Out of this, his technique was born.

Dr. Whitcomb treated people suffering from fibromyalgia from all across the world at his Lake Tahoe clinic, getting astounding results (although not helping everybody). A typical treatment program consisted of ten weeks of care, after which the patient went home with no follow-up care. This resulted in some patients becoming sick again, which naturally caused a lot of backlash.

Dr. Whitcomb was very successful and drew a lot of attention. However, some of his patients who relapsed took to the Internet to voice their unhappiness, and more and more attention started to be focused on Dr. Whitcomb and his Lake Tahoe clinic. After some negative media attention, Dr. Whitcomb was finally brought before the California chiropractic board, eventually losing his chiropractic license. Please note that while he was found guilty of several charges, including excessive treatment plans (above industry standards), advertising violations, failure to provide adequate structural examinations, and failure to perform follow-up examinations, his technique itself was never faulted by the board.

I have personally met Dr. Whitcomb and found him to be pleasant, humble, and deeply passionate about helping people suffering from fibromyalgia. Unfortunately, controversy still surrounds his name today, and opponents of his work are very vocal. Because of this, his work almost stopped when he left practice.

Thankfully, David Singer, DC, a well-known chiropractic practice management coach, saved this technique from certain death after he discovered it and made it available to other health care professionals. The technique was tweaked somewhat (although not much) and doctors were taught proper record-keeping and careful, supportive follow-up care with each patient. Today, this work is used by doctors all around the world, as far as the Netherlands and Australia, with astounding results. In my office, it is one of the best tools in my arsenal. I have seen great outcomes with the neurological symptoms associated with fibromyalgia and other conditions such as RSD/CRPS (reflex sympathetic dystrophy, or chronic regional pain syndrome).

Before a patient enters treatment with this upper cervical technique, the patient is tested first to see if they are a good candidate for treatment. This test consists of gentle pressure applied in a specific manner to the upper cervical spine. If the patient has the neurological symptoms associated with some cases of fibromyalgia caused by cervical trauma or stenosis, their pain will most often notably and dramatically decrease (although temporarily) while this pressure is applied. This lets the doctor know that the patient will most likely respond favorably to care. The treatment itself consists of a series of very specific adjustments to the upper cervical spine over a certain prescribed period of time. Please note that the patient's response to this test cannot be predicted by failure to obtain results through previous chiropractic adjustments. In other words, even if chiropractic didn't work for you in the past, you may still respond to this one specific technique.

While ongoing research is still needed, it is theorized that this treatment decreases meningeal compression. The meninges are three layers that surround the brain and spinal cord and can become trapped, pulled, or compressed after neck or head trauma. It is also my opinion that this technique causes a massive normalizing shift of the autonomic or automatic nervous system. This often results in the patient feeling almost euphoric and very relaxed during and immediately after the test. I have made a dramatic difference in many patients' lives using this work as one of my tools, and I highly recommend it if you are suffering from fibromyalgia.

You can see if there is a doctor near you using this work by going to www.nrc.md and plugging in your zip code.

CHAPTER 6

OTHER POSSIBLE CULPRITS

The last straw breaks the camel's back.
—English proverb

Everything in excess is opposed to nature.
—Hippocrates

Not every single patient with fibromyalgia will suffer from an old neck injury or stenosis. Many other factors may contribute to the onset of it. Additionally, it's possible for more than one factor to combine and finally reach critical mass, which in turn triggers the onset of fibromyalgia in the patient. This chapter discusses some more possible culprits.

TOXICITY

Why does your house get messy? There are two possible reasons, or usually a combination of both. The first reason is that you are too busy or overwhelmed to clean it. Things get put off (like vacuuming or folding laundry) and pile up. The other reason it may get messy is that you can't keep up with it, since it's being messed up faster than you can clean (if you have children, you probably know what I mean). Think of your body as a house. Every day, toxins enter your body and your "house" gets dirty.

WHAT ARE TOXINS?

Toxins can enter our bodies from the external environment or be produced by us internally. Our body naturally produces internal toxins as a by-product of the metabolic functions it performs each day. Antioxidants are crucial in eliminating free radicals from your body. What exactly are free radicals? Free radicals are basically very reactive particles (small loose cannons, if you will) that move all around the cell damaging everything they come in contact with. Most are produced as a by-product of metabolism, but they can also arise from exposure to toxins, such as heavy metals.

In a nutshell, we are bombarded by toxins. When the body digests food, it produces toxins and waste. When it heals and repairs itself, it produces waste. Whenever we experience negative feelings like stress or anger, we also produce harmful toxins.

However, our bodies were designed to be able to naturally eliminate these toxins. We get into trouble when we are bombarded with the second kind of toxins, which are found in our food, water, and environment: human-made toxins. We eat them, drink them, breathe them, touch them, inject them, swallow them in our medications, and put them on our skins regularly and repeatedly. Our cells never get a break! We live in a toxic environment, and while you can control some aspects of your environment (such as the food you eat) it is impossible to avoid toxins altogether.

Consider this: according to the Environmental Protection Agency (EPA), four billion pounds of chemicals are released into the ground and hundreds of millions of pounds of chemicals discharged into surface waters such as lakes and rivers each year. In the United States we allow more than ten thousand additives into our food supply.

Americans each eat an average of about one hundred and forty-two pounds of additives and toxins each year. Typically, eight pounds come from salt, one hundred and twenty pounds come from sugar, and about fourteen pounds from coloring, preservatives, and flavorings. It is not a question of "if" we are toxic, but rather of how much it affects our health.

The body gets rid of toxins through breathing and sweating as well as through the colon, kidneys, and liver. When my patients mention a detox, they are most often thinking of a colon detox. However, the liver is incredibly overburdened and must not be ignored. Why may your liver be overworked? The liver performs over five hundred different tasks and is truly an amazing organ. However, your liver is essentially the filter of your bloodstream, and like any filter, it can become clogged with waste materials when it takes in more toxins than it can filter. When toxins overwhelm the liver, it can no longer perform as it should. Fat may accumulate in the liver or in other organs. Toxins build up and get into the bloodstream.

Among the signs of a toxic liver are weight gain (especially around the abdomen), headaches, bloating, indigestion, high blood pressure, elevated cholesterol, food allergies, memory loss, fatigue, acne, mood swings, depression, and even skin rashes. When the liver cannot do its work, the toxins that we are exposed to accumulate in the body and make us ill in an assortment of ways. They have damaging effects on many body functions, particularly the immune system. An overworked and undernourished liver is recognized as the root cause of many chronic diseases.

HEAVY METALS

Heavy metals include lead, mercury, cadmium, antimony, aluminum, arsenic, and many others. Many of the heavy metals, such as zinc, copper, chromium, iron, and manganese, are essential to body function in very small amounts. But if these metals accumulate in the body in concentrations sufficient to cause poisoning, serious damage may occur. Heavy metals enter our bodies in many ways. They may enter through cosmetics, amalgam dental fillings, water, improperly coated food containers and cookware, vaccinations, cigarettes, and many other things in our environment.

Symptoms of heavy metal poisoning include anemia, fatigue, musculoskeletal complaints, mood disturbances, neurological problems, high blood pressure, gastrointestinal (GI) symptoms, kidney problems, liver dysfunction, endocrine problems, hormonal imbalances, and immune system dysfunction. Heavy metal toxicity causes systemic problems that may fit the symptoms of many other syndromes. It presents in various body systems, depending on where the biochemical imbalance or disruption occurs, or the area(s) of highest concentrations of the metal(s)—for example, the brain, kidneys, or pituitary. Long-term exposure may contribute to the onset of slow progressive conditions such as Alzheimer's disease, Parkinson's disease, and cancer.

Laboratory tests routinely used for exposed persons include blood tests, liver and renal function tests, urine tests, fecal tests, X-rays, and hair and fingernail analyses. Many of these tests are not routinely performed in your doctor's office, but you should be able to find a doctor who can perform a urine test. While it is widely assumed that hair or fingernail analyses are best, I prefer urine analysis. Hair and fingernail analyses can give an indication of exposure that has occurred over time or in the past but will not show recent exposures. It may also give false positives. Blood will only reflect recent and severe exposure. In addition, the body does not use blood as a detoxifying pathway, but it does use urine as such. Urine will reflect exposures that are chronic or that have happened in the last few days.

Heavy metal detoxification may be done in many ways. Many health care professionals use chelating agents. These include:

- **Dimercaptosuccinic acid (DMSA)**, which, although being FDA-approved, is mostly not recommended due to severe possible side effects, as well as unpredictable redistribution of mercury after being pulled from the kidneys, causing the mercury to be redeposited in the brain, kidneys, liver, or muscle tissue.

- **Ethylenediaminetetraacetic acid (EDTA)**, which is not a natural supplement. Like DMSA, EDTA is FDA-approved. It has traditionally been used to treat lead poisoning. Unlike DMSA, EDTA is a weak chelator of mercury. Taking EDTA can be dangerous because it will chelate calcium and other essential minerals out of the body along with the toxic heavy metals.

- **Dimercapto-propane sulfonate (DMPS)**, an experimental drug used for chelation, not approved by the FDA. Some doctors question the safety of this drug, pointing to the lack of research on its long-term effects on the human body.

- **Chlorella**, a variety of algae found in fresh water such as ponds or lakes. It is commonly used as a natural chelation supplement, meaning that it pulls out heavy metals such as mercury from the body. However, chlorella also pulls mercury from the water it is grown in, which naturally defeats the purpose of taking it in the first place. Analysis of at least one specimen of commercially available chlorella has shown high levels of mercury. You don't want to take a supplement riddled with mercury in order to remove mercury; that doesn't make sense.

- **Zeolite**, volcanic rock that attracts toxins and physically removes them from the body. Think of it as a taxi, loading up all the bad guys. Zeolite has a negative charge and a "honeycomb" structure with lots of holes. It is thought that this negative charge acts like a magnet and pulls the positively charged toxins, especially toxic metals, into the cells of the honeycomb, where the trapped toxins are then eliminated from the body through urine, sweat, and feces. Some animal studies have shown promise, and it is not a harmful substance, although some good minerals may be pulled from the body using zeolite. Mineral supplementation is recommended while using this product.

- **The ionic foot detox**, a footbath with an electric current. In a typical session the patient places their feet in warm salt water and an electrical array is turned on, creating electrolysis in the water. This electrolysis causes an electromagnetic field in the water that pulls toxins and heavy metals into the water through the sweat glands in the feet. During the session, the water changes color and small floating particles appear. Although many people claim that the color change of the water is due to oxidation only and that this method is a hoax, the truth is that 60 percent of the color change of the water is due to oxidation, and the other 40 percent is, in fact, due to the individual patient's toxicity, and will vary depending on the patient. I have personally seen notable and immediate reactions in my practice to this footbath, and I not only use it as part of my treatment plan, but I also use it personally twice a week.

- **Fasting and dietary detoxification**, generally consisting of cutting down on the number of calories you take in, eating very pure foods (consisting of lean organic grass-fed protein, raw nuts, and fruits and vegetables only, or juicing fruits and vegetables, or fasting and drinking lots of water). The general approach here is to provide the body with good nutrition while forcing it into ketosis, the process by which it is essentially burning its own fat for fuel. When the liver is overwhelmed, it does what any tired employee does—it puts its work off for later, to be detoxified when the liver isn't quite so busy. The body does this by depositing the harmful toxins in fat, sort of like a messy storage room. This protects the body and its valuable organs from these free-floating toxins. However, for many of us, those days of detoxification never comes. When we fast, or reduce our calorie intake, the body will burn this dirty fat, and that day of reckoning and processing all those old toxins will finally arrive.

HEAVY METAL/CANDIDA LINK

If you suffer from fibromyalgia and you have researched possible solutions on the Internet or elsewhere, no doubt have you have come across the possible benefits of treating a candida or yeast overgrowth in the body. Candida albicans is a parasitic fungus that normally occurs in the gut, vagina, mouth, and other areas of the body.

Usually, candida is kept in check by your body's friendly or good bacteria. However, when the body is not well or when we take antibiotics that kill our friendly bacteria, this parasite will grow too rapidly and we may suffer from a host of different unpleasant symptoms, such as allergies, fatigue, sugar cravings, itching and burning, skin rashes, and many more. Candida can also damage the gut, leading to leaky gut syndrome. This will cause large particles to enter the bloodstream, in turn leading to autoimmune conditions and allergies (such as gluten intolerance) and affecting the brain and nervous system.

There are a variety of ways to kill a candida overgrowth in the body, one of which is to simply build up the body's good bacteria again. It is a very difficult infection to treat; it may take many months to get it under control in severe cases. However, a somewhat unknown but crucial piece of the candida puzzle that *must not* be ignored is possible heavy metal toxicity. How are they linked?

Candida yeast serves the purpose of absorbing and sequestering heavy metals. Yeast overgrowth is one of the body's defenses to try and keep mercury and other heavy metals from damaging body tissues such as the brain. In other words, candida absorbs and binds mercury, thus protecting your body. As mentioned before, your body is infinitely smart. In its wisdom, it will choose a symbiotic relationship with the candida parasite over mercury toxicity. While candida is unhealthy, it is not as immediately damaging as mercury. Therefore, the body is choosing the lesser of two evils. When the uninformed patient or health care professional then embarks on a war against candida, massive amounts of free mercury are released into the body, causing much more harm than good. If you suffer from a suspected candida overgrowth, it is therefore *crucial* that you get tested and treated for heavy metal toxicity first. Be especially diligent if you have or have ever had amalgam fillings in your teeth.

THE DANGER IN YOUR MOUTH

Besides flossing, brushing our teeth, and getting professionally checked and cleaned a few times a year if we are diligent, most of us don't give our teeth a second thought.

I was first introduced to the importance of teeth while studying biological medicine. Biological medicine recognizes that the human being is a part of nature and reacts like everything else in nature. It seeks to awaken the healing powers that lie within us all through the use of natural methods and remedies. I was introduced to this work by one of my mentors, Thomas Rau, MD.

Dr. Rau is the medical director at the world's largest privately owned clinic, the Paracelsus clinic (www.Paracelsus.ch). The Paracelsus clinic is located an hour away from Zurich, Switzerland, and employs about a hundred doctors, half of whom are dentists. People from all over the world come to this clinic to be treated for cancer, autoimmune conditions, and other conditions, often with astounding, unprecedented success.

Dr. Rau taught me that the teeth are linked to energy meridians, further linked to every organ in your body. It is crucial that the mouth be healthy. There is a reason why almost half the medical staff at this groundbreaking clinic are dentists. When patients enter care at the Paracelsus clinic, their mouths are carefully examined.

Here are a few things that could be of concern in the mouth:

AMALGAM FILLINGS

If you have any silver-colored fillings in your mouth, this is usually a bad sign. A typical amalgam filling consists of approximately 50 percent mercury and 30 percent silver, as well as tin and copper. Mercury is a powerful poison. Published research demonstrates that mercury is more toxic than lead, cadmium, or arsenic. No amount of exposure to mercury vapor can be considered harmless, especially considering its cumulative effect.

In spite of numerous published scientific studies over the years demonstrating the ill effects of mercury fillings in the mouth, and considering that the FDA has never approved the amalgam mixture as a safe dental device, mercury/silver/amalgam fillings are still the primary material used by dentists in the United States (approximately one hundred million fillings are performed yearly).

The American Dental Association maintains that mercury is safe to use and harmless in the mouth, as the mixing of mercury is supposed to "bind" the mercury safely and render it harmless. However, electron microscopes have shown tiny droplets of mercury on the surface of amalgam fillings. Also, mercury vapors have been proven to escape these fillings and enter the blood stream. Meanwhile, the World Health Organization has concluded that dental fillings contribute more mercury to the human body than all other sources combined.

Let's just ignore the controversy and look at a few facts about mercury: Mercury, before it is placed into the mouth, is a recognized hazardous toxin. The scrap amalgam that is removed from the mouth cannot simply be thrown away in the trash, or the dentist may be subject to a ten-thousand-dollar fine by the Environmental Protection Agency (EPA). Instead, the scrap is considered a toxic waste and must be removed by a hazardous waste company in a specific way to keep the mercury from entering the water system.

It is crucial, if you have these fillings removed, that you have it done by an experienced dentist, as the removal is tricky and if done incorrectly may do more harm than good. Often the body is flooded with mercury during the removal process.

ROOT CANALS

A root canal is a common dental procedure that nearly every dentist will assure you is completely safe, despite the fact that scientists have been warning of its dangers for more than a hundred years. More than twenty-five million root canals are performed every year in this country.

Every day in the United States alone, approximately forty-one thousand of these dental procedures are performed on patients who believe they are safely and permanently fixing their problem. Sadly, the vast majority of dentists are oblivious to the serious potential health risks they are exposing their patients to, risks that persist for the rest of their patients' lives. The American Dental Association claims root canals have been proven safe, but they have no published data or actual research to substantiate their claim.

Teeth that have undergone root canals are dead teeth that can become dangerous incubators for highly toxic anaerobic bacteria.

These bacteria could make their way into your bloodstream to cause a number of serious medical conditions, many of which might not appear until many years later. A tooth has one to four major canals. This is what is taught in dental school, and what is cleaned out in root canals. What is lesser known and often ignored by dentists and dental schools are the additional "accessory canals." A doctor named Weston Price did extensive research on these.

Dr. Price (1870–1948) was a dentist known primarily for his theories on the relationship between nutrition, dental health, and physical health. Dr. Price identified as many as seventy-five separate accessory canals in a single central incisor or front tooth. When we look at the structure of a tooth, we find three layers. First is the outer layer, known as enamel; then comes the second layer, known as dentin; and the inner part is the pulp chamber where the nerve resides. On the outside of the tooth is a ligament called the periodontal ligament, formed by fibers that come out of the tooth and intertwine with fibers coming out of the bone. Teeth are not actually attached directly to bone, but are attached by this ligament.

The second layer of the tooth, the dentin, is not really solid but composed of tiny tubules or canals. In a front tooth, if all these tubules were attached end to end, they would reach over three miles. Note that the tubules have adequate space to house many thousands of bacteria. Most of these toxic teeth feel and look fine for many years, which makes their role in systemic disease even harder to trace back. In addition, these dead teeth may cause secondary infections in the bones of the jaw and face, not easily detected by the untrained eye on X-ray.

Many other problems can stem from teeth, such as other toxic materials or metals used in dental work, gum disease and infection, and the mixture of incompatible metals, such as gold fillings with certain metal fillings. If you suffer from fibromyalgia, cancer, or other chronic conditions, I urge you to have your teeth examined by a trained biological or holistic dentist.

The following organizations can help you to find a mercury-free, biological dentist:

- Consumers for Dental Choice

- International Academy of Biological Dentistry & Medicine (IABDM)

- Holistic Dental Association

- International Association of Mercury-Safe Dentists

FIBROMYALGIA PATIENTS BEWARE!

When it comes to patients suffering from fibromyalgia, it is *very* important that great caution be taken when detoxifying. Even for a healthy individual, detoxification is very hard on all the organs and can cause symptoms such as headaches, muscle aches, fatigue, diarrhea, nausea, tremors, crying fits and anger, and many other side effects.

People who suffer from fibromyalgia are especially vulnerable to the side effects of detoxification, and their bodies are not always equipped to handle the stress of it. Often, well-meaning health professionals will detoxify fibromyalgia patients immediately after they start care in an effort to decrease their pain and increase their chances of healing. However, unless the fibromyalgia patient's nervous system and body are strong enough to tolerate the side effects of detoxification, it will often do more harm than good. In my clinic, I do not attempt to detoxify fibromyalgia patients until their neurological symptoms are at least 75 percent decreased.

We recommend that you only embark on a detoxification program with the help of a health professional experienced not only in detoxification, but also in fibromyalgia. Make sure that they have had success in the past and, when possible, ask if you can personally speak to some of their past fibromyalgia patients who have had positive results, with their permission. Also know that detoxification may alter the effects of the prescription medications you take and should be monitored.

Your medical doctor, while responsible for monitoring the medication you are taking and its effects on your body, will typically be unfamiliar with the detoxification process, as most medical doctors are not trained in this area. Your doctor may often tell you not to bother with it, since a lot of alternative and unknown things may make your doctor nervous and suspicious. Again, you have to be your own advocate; make sure that you are comfortable with the detoxification process and its proven success, and make sure you know what to expect and its side effects. The golden rule for *any* detoxification in the fibromyalgia patient is: slow and easy does it.

AUTOIMMUNE CONDITIONS: WHEN YOUR BODY TURNS ON ITSELF

Our immune system is like a complex army of special cells that act like soldiers. Together with our organs, it defends the body from germs, viruses, and other foreign invaders. As with any army, it is vitally important that your immune system be able to tell the enemy from its own soldiers—the self from the non-self. In autoimmune conditions, the body has lost this ability. When this happens, the body makes antibodies that turn on it with deadly precision and mistakenly attack normal cells. At the same time, special cells called regulatory T-cells (the army majors) fail to do their job of keeping the immune system in line. The result is a misguided and very devastating attack on your own body. This causes the damage we know as autoimmune disease. The body parts that are affected depend on the type of autoimmune disease. There are more than eighty known types of autoimmune conditions and diseases.

THE NERVOUS SYSTEM'S ROLE

Once again, we return to the role of the nervous system and the fact that it does not appear to be functioning correctly in the fibromyalgia patient. This also negatively affects the immune system. Clear links have been established between the nervous system and the immune system. There is ongoing communication between the "soldiers" or cells involved in the immune response and the nervous system.[19] The chemicals that convey messages among nerve cells also communicate with the cells of the immune system. If the nervous system is disorganized, the immune system becomes confused and is unable to tell the non-self from the self.

While fibromyalgia is not classified as an autoimmune condition, patients who suffer from fibromyalgia will often develop autoimmune conditions such as allergies, rheumatoid arthritis (RA), Hashimoto's thyroiditis (a condition where the thyroid gland is attacked by the body's own immune system), systemic lupus erythematosus (a long-term autoimmune disorder where the body attacks its own organs and joints), Sjögren's syndrome (a chronic autoimmune disease in which the white blood cells attack the moisture-producing glands), and many others.

It is my belief that all patients suffering from fibromyalgia should be routinely screened for autoimmune conditions. The fact that their nervous systems are essentially not communicating with their immune systems makes them much more vulnerable to these conditions.

FOOD ALLERGIES

The body can respond to food to which it is allergic in two ways: right away and later. This is also known as immediate and delayed responses. True allergies to food are different than sensitivity or intolerance to certain foods, like lactose intolerance. Allergic reactions are true immune responses with potentially far-reaching negative effects on the entire body. The immediate reactions are those that people are usually aware they have, and are quite noticeable. Such reactions occur within a few hours after eating the offending food, and may include a rash, or difficulty breathing in severe cases (anaphylactic shock).

It is easy to make a correlation with how one feels after eating a specific food if the reaction is very noticeable and almost immediate. On the other hand, a delayed reaction may not occur for a few hours to even a few days after eating the food. It is not uncommon for a person to drink a glass of milk today, for example, and have an asthma attack or rash tomorrow, never connecting their symptoms to the milk. It is these kinds of delayed reactions that often go undetected. They may affect people's health and lives for years, sometimes a whole lifetime, without being identified. When food allergies are identified and properly treated, the relief can greatly improve a person's health.

It has been observed that up to 60 percent of fibromyalgia patients suffer from one or more allergies.[20] If the fibromyalgia patient eats food that he or she is allergic to, it will cause an inflammatory reaction within the body (think of a sunburn inside the body), which will increase the severity of the pain and symptoms. The continued and prolonged release of histamines may cause brain fog and widespread pain and aching in the body. While it is my belief that food allergies rarely cause fibromyalgia, I do believe that they often develop in fibromyalgia sufferers and increase their misery. They are fuel that feeds the fibromyalgia fire.

Fibromyalgia patients may develop food allergies for several reasons. Once again, one must view the body as one organism in which each malfunctioning part affects the entire body. In a fibromyalgia patient, the central nervous system is not functioning correctly, and this in turn causes the immune system to act improperly when introduced to some common foods. The other link between fibromyalgia and food allergies is an improperly functioning GI (gastrointestinal) system. While the GI system will be discussed in great detail in chapter 10 , I do want to address leaky gut syndrome here.

LEAKY GUT AND ALLERGIES

Patients who suffer from intestinal disorders, such as a leaky gut, will often develop allergies.[21] What exactly is a leaky gut? Normally, the intestinal lining forms a barrier between all the stuff we eat and our blood. This protects our bodies and also filters needed nutrients from unwanted ones. The small intestine is designed to allow very small particles of digested nutrients to pass through its wall and into the bloodstream, where it is distributed throughout the body as needed.

Due to a variety of causes, the intestinal wall can become more permeable or "leaky" and allow larger, half-digested food particles or toxins and waste to pass through, causing what is known as leaky gut syndrome. The cause of this may be decreased nervous system communication to the gut, resulting in "bad housekeeping" and damage to the gut, which is often the case in fibromyalgia. Other possible causes may be chronic inflammation, using the birth control pill, chronic emotional stress, food sensitivities, a sluggish liver, damage from taking large amounts of nonsteroidal anti-inflammatory drugs (NSAIDS), medications, radiation or certain antibiotics, excessive and long-term alcohol, caffeine, or tobacco use, too much sugar, heavy metal toxicity, candida overgrowth, or decreased immunity.

When these particles enter the bloodstream, the immune system recognizes them as foreign invaders and attempts to fight them off. Over a long period of time, this will cause your immune system to malfunction and may result in autoimmune conditions and allergies. The first step in treating leaky gut syndrome and other GI problems in a fibromyalgia patient should be restoring proper nervous system communication to the GI system, as discussed later in this book.

PERIMENOPAUSE

Perimenopause, or the period of transition into menopause, is the stage of a female's reproductive life that begins several years before menopause, when the ovaries gradually begin to produce less estrogen. It usually starts in a woman's forties, but can start in her thirties or even earlier. Perimenopause will usually last about four years, but its onset may also be very short (a few months) and sudden, surprising and confusing the woman in whose body it is taking place. Perimenopause ends in menopause, at which point the ovaries stop releasing eggs. This transition from perimenopause into full-blown menopause is usually a gradual one. In the last one or two years of perimenopause, the decline in estrogen greatly accelerates. At this stage, many women may experience menopausal symptoms.

Perimenopause may cause great stress in the female body. Keep in mind, *any* change in the internal environment of our bodies is naturally stressful, since it requires adaptation and change. Women who suffer from fibromyalgia have been shown to have neuroendocrine (involving the nerve stimulation of various glands) abnormalities,[22] making any hormonal changes especially stressful for their bodies. Perimenopause and menopause may also *mimic* fibromyalgia to some extent, and should always be ruled out before fibromyalgia is diagnosed. When fibromyalgia collides with these periods of transition, it may exacerbate the fibromyalgia symptoms and can make the woman feel incredibly sore, exhausted, and irritable. Menopause often makes your muscles ache, since muscles often hurt and feel sore due to hormonal changes. Sleep loss from menopause and changing hormones can also make you achy, adding to the sleep deprivation that fibromyalgia is so notorious for.

Many women are diagnosed with fibromyalgia right as they enter perimenopause or menopause. If you understand that perimenopause and menopause cause great biochemical changes in the female body, it makes sense that perimenopause or menopause will often trigger fibromyalgia in itself. Remember that physical, chemical, and emotional stress pile up until they reach a critical point, at which time any number of different conditions or symptoms, like fibromyalgia, can rear their ugly heads.

I am personally opposed to synthetic hormone replacement therapy (HRT), due to its unnatural and invasive effect on the body and its potentially serious side effects, such as increased blood clotting, increased risk of certain cancers, high blood pressure, and pancreatitis. However, since we live in a highly toxic world, our hormonal balances are often not ideal. Many toxins will disrupt our endocrine system, such as cosmetic products, pesticides, and medications. For this reason, we suggest that any patient suffering from fibromyalgia seek out the guidance of a health care practitioner experienced in *natural* hormone replacement therapy.

Phytotherapy (the use of plants in treating symptoms) has long been a gentle approach to a complex issue, where herbs like wild yam, black cohosh, ashwagandha, and chasteberry are used to restore hormonal balance. While patients often assume that it is the mere absence of estrogen wreaking havoc in the menopausal or post-hysterectomy patient, the importance of the overall delicate *balance* between hormones, such as progesterone, estrogen, and testosterone is often overlooked and must be addressed. Keep in mind that your fat cells actually produce estrogen.

In addition, a fibromyalgia patient should limit exposure to xenoestrogens (unnatural, industrial compounds and toxins that have estrogen-like effects on the body). Try to use organic beauty products and cosmetics, limit your exposure to pesticides as much as possible, try to eat a natural, organic diet whenever possible, and restore your internal health with smart supplementation (read the supplementation chapter elsewhere in this book.)

VESTIBULAR INJURIES

Chances are you have never heard of a vestibular injury. This is a pretty unknown injury to the inner ear, and the chances that the average allopathic doctor or alternative doctor will diagnose you with it are pretty slim. Although a vestibular injury does not start out as fibromyalgia, it is often *confused* with fibromyalgia in its early stages. However, if this condition remains untreated, it will often progress and the patient will develop fibromyalgia. Therefore, I consider it one of the possible causes of fibromyalgia. If you suffer from dizziness and anxiety and cannot stand elevators or large stores with no windows (like Costco or Sam's club), you may suffer from vestibular symptoms. Please go to http://vestibular.org/ understanding-vestibular-disorder/symptoms for more information.

OXYGEN DEPRIVATION

Oxygen deprivation is often a trigger or contributor to fibromyalgia. Causes of oxygen deprivation include asthma as well as conditions that may cause fibrosis of the lungs, such as ankylosing spondylitis (degenerative arthritis that affects primarily the spine) or interstitial lung disease (ILD). ILD describes any disorder that causes scarring of the lung, such as asbestos exposure or autoimmune diseases.

Another possible culprit is carbon monoxide poisoning. When oxygen is poorly metabolized, it may cause fatigue and pain in muscles, memory disruption in the brain, and impaired function of all of our body's cells. Oxygen metabolism (the process of successfully delivering oxygen to each cell in the body) may also be affected by long-term oxidative stress on the inside of the body (think of an old car that is rusting), caused by a sugar overload, excessive antibiotics, toxins, allergies, a poor diet, or bad fats.

Majid Ali, MD, has done a lot of research in this field. He describes oxygen-deprivation fibromyalgia patients as "human canaries."

Canaries were (sadly if you love cute birds) used until the 1980s to detect low oxygen levels in coal mines, since they continuously sing. When a caged canary was taken down a coalmine and stopped singing, toxic levels of carbon monoxide were suspected in the mine. Sometimes, it's not so much a question of low oxygen available to the cells, but an inability of the body to *use* the oxygen available.

In carbon monoxide poisoning, a free radical called nitric oxide is released by cells as a waste product in response to the poisoning. It is a powerful vasodilator, meaning that the body will release this chemical in response to low oxygen levels to dilate the vascular system in order to get more oxygen to the organs in danger of dying. This waste product will injure the body chemically and may lead to the critical mass of stress that can result in the symptoms of fibromyalgia.

Patients suffering from oxygen deprivation may benefit from hyperbaric chamber therapy, detoxification, and supplementation (to increase oxygen levels in the cells). Please look at the supplementation chapter elsewhere in this book (chapter 9).

SLEEP APNEA

Sleep apnea is a common condition in which you stop breathing for short periods of time while sleeping and/or take very shallow breaths while you sleep. These pauses in breathing can last from a few seconds to many minutes. They may occur dozens of times an hour. Typically, after these short periods where you stop breathing, normal breathing resumes again, sometimes with a loud noise, snore, or choking sound. Basically, the brain forgets to tell the body to breathe. In self-defense, the body will wake you up, forcing you to take over manual control of your breathing again.

Sleep apnea is usually a chronic condition that disrupts a person's rest over a long period of time. When breathing becomes shallower or pauses, the apnea sufferer will often move out of deep (REM) sleep into light sleep. As a result, the quality of sleep is quite poor, which makes the apnea sufferer chronically tired and affects the person's immune system, concentration, and healing. One study found that while this did not appear to affect many women suffering from fibromyalgia, at least 44 percent of all males with fibromyalgia suffered from sleep apnea.[23] Other estimates put this number as high as 60 percent for males.

EMOTIONAL STRESS

Prolonged or intense emotional stress may trigger the development of fibromyalgia and almost always contributes, at least partially, to its cause. Several studies have, in fact, proved that emotional stress may directly cause fibromyalgia.[24, 25] When the brain perceives a threat, the nervous system will respond as if your survival is being threatened. The body responds by releasing stress hormones such as cortisol, which has many negative effects on the body, such as weight gain in the stomach area, increase in "bad" cholesterol, and high blood pressure. It may also contribute to the cascade of events that eventually bring a patient to the point where they exhibit the symptoms of fibromyalgia. To better understand how stress affects your nervous system and contributes to the neurological symptoms of fibromyalgia, make sure you read the chapter on autonomic dysfunction later in this book.

SOME COMBINATION OF TWO OR MORE TYPES

It is rare that one single cause, besides cervical injury, is responsible for the development of fibromyalgia; rather, it is typically a combination of different factors. It's important to identify which factors contributed to your poor health, and to systematically address and correct each one to the best of your ability.

CHAPTER 7

THE MONKEY ON YOUR BACK: UNDERSTANDING THE AUTONOMIC NERVOUS SYSTEM AND HOW IT CAN MAKE YOU SICK

It is not the strongest of the species that survives, nor the most intelligent that survives. It is the one that is the most adaptable to change.
—Charles Darwin

I promise you nothing is as chaotic as it seems. Nothing is worth your health. Nothing is worth poisoning yourself into stress, anxiety, and fear.
—Steve Maraboli

The nervous system holds the key to the body's incredible potential to heal itself.
—Sir Jay Holder, MD, DC, PhD

> *We have not found a way to reverse the fight-or-flight dominance in fibromyalgia permanently. Once we find that, I think we will have discovered the cure to fibromyalgia. The best we can do for now is treat the problems caused by fight-or-flight dominance and try and encourage the nervous system to shift into rest-and-digest mode whenever possible.*
> —G. Liptan, MD

In this chapter, we take a closer look at the autonomic (or automatic) nervous system. While I don't need you to become an expert on neurology (who has the time?), I do want to make sure that you have a good basic understanding of how this system works and what it controls (everything!) so that many of the mysterious neurological symptoms associated with fibromyalgia will make sense to you. When you understand how something started going haywire in the first place, you can begin the process of fixing it.

Typically, our current health care system consists of managing symptoms. This can be done in many different ways. Nerve signals of pain and discomfort are seen as a bothersome and unwanted symptom and may be numbed or interrupted. Nerves may be removed. Organs will also often be removed. If a part hurts, it must be silenced, numbed, or taken out. Today, this way of thinking has become normal for most of us.

What I am about to say may sound extreme, but I stand by it. Unless the body is in an emergency situation where immediate action is needed to prevent permanent damage, organ loss, or death, medical management of symptoms rarely contributes to improved health, and most often may actually take away from the patient's overall quality of life. Please note that under some circumstances, such as Parkinson's, symptom management is very understandable and appropriate. However, generally speaking, symptom management should preferably be exercised only for limited periods of time.

All that being said, it's understandable *why* fibromyalgia sufferers reach for relief in a bottle. It is impossible to function in everyday life while in excruciating pain. However, such management of pain should never be confused with a healing process or improved health. Please note that I do not judge anyone who reaches for pain relief. My hope is simply for you to find the answers that will make it possible for you to live without daily pain medication.

Let's take a closer look at the autonomic nervous system and how it may cause some of the most common symptoms associated with fibromyalgia.

YOUR AUTOPILOT GONE WRONG

What if your body was an airplane and your pilot drunk? The autonomic nervous system (sometimes known as the automatic or involuntary nervous system) is incredibly important to your health, as this system is the master control system that runs every single function in your body. Most of these functions require no conscious thought from you. You don't have to remember to breathe, for example. When you are sitting in an airplane, you don't have to know exactly what the pilot is doing up there in the cabin. You just trust that he is doing his job and will keep the plane in the air and eventually land it safely. In the case of most fibromyalgia sufferers, the pilot is unfortunately up to all sorts of monkey business, and usually has his hand frozen in the full-throttle position.

I definitely do not want to bore you with the anatomy and physiology of the nervous system. It was painful enough for me to learn it. However, in the spirit of understanding fibromyalgia, I do briefly want to explain how it is put together. The autonomic nervous system is the part of the nervous system outside of the central nervous system (the brain and the spinal cord) that acts as a control system, functioning largely without any conscious effort from you. This system is further divided into two systems: the sympathetic nervous system (SNS) and the parasympathetic nervous system (PSNS). It controls many functions such as breathing, heart rate, digestion, sweating, saliva secretion, perspiration, eye dilation, urination, and sexual arousal.

The sympathetic and parasympathetic nervous systems have exactly opposite effects on the functions of the body. They essentially work in opposition to each other, but in a way that complements each other. The balance between the two is *crucial* for the perfect function of every cell in your body. If your body were a car, the sympathetic nervous system would be the gas pedal, and the parasympathetic nervous system would be the brake. While they are both crucial to the car, they cannot be stepped on at the same time. In the typical fibromyalgia syndrome patient, the sympathetic nervous system has its pedal to the metal, all the time. And, as many fibromyalgia sufferers unfortunately find out firsthand, this is bad news for your health. The golden rule of the autonomic nervous system is that if one system is up, the other system must be down.

THE SYMPATHETIC NERVOUS SYSTEM:

"Fight or flight"

This system was designed to help your body fight to stay alive when your survival is being threatened. Think of a caveman in hand-to-paw combat with a saber-toothed tiger. This portion of your nervous system responds very quickly (think zero to ninety in a few seconds), since one usually doesn't have time to calmly ponder one's response to a life-threatening situation. When your life is being threatened and your body gets ready to fight in order to ensure its survival, every small bit of energy spent is carefully considered. Nothing is wasted. Energy will be rerouted away from systems that do not concern themselves with short-term survival, to where it can be used more readily to fight an immediate threat. For example, blood will flow away from the digestive tract and skin in order to be rationed out to the lungs and muscles. It is more important under those circumstances to be able to fight using your muscles, and to breathe hard and fast, as your body needs oxygen.

Speaking of oxygen, the bronchioles (small air passages) in the lungs will open up, which allows for more oxygen into the blood. At the same time the heart will beat faster. Another physiological change in the body is that the pupils will dilate, allowing more light to enter the eyes. The adrenal glands on top of the kidneys will pump adrenalin in case you need extra motivation besides fear to fight. It will also make all the sphincters (think of pressure valves) in the body, like the urinary sphincter, contract and close tight.

So why does this affect you? There probably isn't the equivalent of a saber-toothed tiger chasing you every day. However, your brain cannot distinguish fear and stress from *actual* life-threatening situations. Additionally, as mentioned earlier in this book when we discussed emotional stress, a very old traumatic event can run in a continuous "loop" in the subconscious mind. The brain cannot distinguish between this old memory and present danger. The old memory almost acts like a computer virus, messing with the software in your nervous system. Your brain does not know that it *isn't happening anymore.*

When a person suffers a neck injury following, for example, a fall or car accident affecting the brainstem directly or indirectly, the sympathetic nervous system will become overexcited, affecting the whole body.[26, 27, 28] This will cause your sympathetic nervous system, or "fight or flight" response, to be stuck in the "on" position day in and day out—and if your sympathetic nervous system is stuck all the time, your parasympathetic nervous system is turned off. This will lead to the classic symptoms of fibromyalgia and other autonomic dysfunction or WAD (whiplash-associated dysfunctions). I will discuss each symptom in detail, after we explain how the parasympathetic nervous system works.

THE PARASYMPATHETIC NERVOUS SYSTEM

"Rest and digest" or "Feed and breed"

Think of your parasympathetic nervous system as the system that calms you down, helps you to rest and sleep, and deals with sexual arousal. It functions to counter the sympathetic system. After a crisis or danger has passed, this system helps to calm the body. Your heart and breathing rates slow, your digestion resumes, your pupils contract, and you stop sweating.

This system will also cause the increase of blood flow to your GI tract following a meal to allow digestion. It stimulates the movements of your intestines (called *peristalsis)* that move food through your intestines. It will constrict the pupil of the eye, cause you to salivate when appropriate, and is responsible for getting you in the mood for sex. This system, if activated, will activate your immune system, cause increased circulation to the skin and extremities, and help to release your "feel-good" hormones, called endorphins. It will also decrease temperature. It is the main control system that promotes healing. This system is usually underactive, suppressed, or turned off in those who suffer from fibromyalgia. No wonder you are not in the mood for getting frisky!

HOW THIS IMBALANCE CAUSES SYMPTOMS

Pain, your dark passenger

There is no symptom more life-robbing to the fibromyalgia sufferer than the constant, widespread, spirit-eroding pain. When you understand the mechanics behind the pain of fibromyalgia, the pain makes perfect sense. Understanding the mechanics of your specific pain will bring you one step closer to hope.

TOXIC LESIONS OF THE DISC(S) IN THE NECK

Since the cervical spine, brain stem, and autonomic nervous system are connected, we should start with the nature of the original injury. When most people picture a disc injury, they think of a disc that was herniated, or "squished," and that will show up as a big red flag on an MRI. Often, patients suffering from fibromyalgia will undergo an MRI to rule out disc problems, because of their neck pain and frequent headaches. It is very common for nothing noteworthy to show up on the X-ray or MRI, and the spine to then be dismissed as a problem. Patients are told that their spinal problems are "normal" for their age, that is, everyone seems to have them at that age. However, spinal degeneration is *never* normal just because it is common.

Sometimes, some of the most devastating disc injuries, in terms of the lingering and destructive effects they have on the body, may go undetected by normal imaging. A study performed on people who died from *non-spinal* injuries following car accidents and had "normal" MRIs and X-rays after these accidents proved this. All these people were found to have disc injuries that had been missed. These injuries included small tears, bulges, and fractures where the vertebra meets the disc.[29]

You may wonder why these small injuries matter. How can such a thing cause fibromyalgia? I credit the developer of a technology I use in my practice called frequency-specific microcurrent (FSM), Carolyn McMakin, MA, DC, for first introducing me to the following information:

Deep inside the discs of the spine (in the "nucleus" of the disc) is a neurotoxic substance called phospholipase A2, or PLA2. A small tear in the cartilage of the disc or in the surrounding parts of the disc will cause PLA2 to leak out into the spinal fluid, thereby exposing the spinal cord to it.

This nasty little substance has been shown to be so neurotoxic and inflammatory when present outside the disc that it will destroy the nerves it comes in contact with. We call this a "toxic lesion" of the spine. The part of the cord most likely to be damaged by this neurotoxic substance (the thalamic tract) just happens to be a part of the spinal cord that carries deep pain information. Usually, because of the location of the disc and this part of the spinal cord, the cord is unfortunately exposed to high levels of PLA2. This causes what is called "central pain," or "thalamic pain," which mimics the pain of fibromyalgia exactly.

Please note: If you have pain or aching in your hands and feet, you need to pay attention here. A very important benchmark of fibromyalgia caused by central pain is aching in the hands and feet.

SUBSTANCE P (THINK P FOR PAIN)

Nerve cells communicate with one another through messengers called "neurotransmitters." Substance P is one of these messengers. It is a protein found in the brain and spinal cord that is associated with some inflammatory processes in the joints. Its function is to cause pain. It essentially sends pain signals to the brain and spinal cord after it receives them from the sensory nerves. Interestingly enough, it has also been shown to be involved in increased stress and anxiety if elevated. The nerves that release Substance P have been shown to most likely be autonomic.[30] Severe or prolonged injury of these autonomic nerves will cause pain in different ways: parts of the spinal cord will become hyperexcitable, making them very sensitive to toxic stimuli, and these in turn will lower the pain threshold in the patient.[31]

Some of the major symptoms of fibromyalgia are easily traced back to the malfunctioning of the autonomic nervous system. As a matter of fact, there are so many common fibromyalgia symptoms related to it that I decided to devote a whole chapter to it.

CHAPTER 8

OF COURSE!
WHEN ALL YOUR SYMPTOMS
START MAKING SENSE

*When you have insomnia, you're never really
asleep...and you're never really awake.*
—Fight Club

God may forgive your sins, but your nervous system won't.
—Alfred Korzybski

SLEEP, A DISTANT MEMORY

The other day I saw a funny T-shirt that reminded me of my fibro-myalgia patients: "Remember when you woke up all refreshed after going to bed early and drifting off to sleep easily? Me either." Besides the constant pain, sleeping problems are probably one of the most annoying and life-robbing symptoms fibromyalgia patients suffer from.

Sleeping serves a very important function. While you are sleeping, your nervous system has much more energy available for healing. There are many reasons for this. During this time, you are not thinking, which might cause you to feel emotions, causing your available energy to be spent on these emotionally loaded thoughts. Your senses are, for the most part, shut down. You are not hearing, seeing, or smelling. You are not using your large muscle groups to move around. All the energy normally used on these functions can now be redirected and used to assist your body in the healing process. However, if you are sleep-deprived, your body is missing out on this golden opportunity. It is estimated that your body heals about three times faster while asleep. It is a cruel twist of fate that the patients who need this healing the most are the very patients who can't sleep.

Sleep problems with fibromyalgia include insomnia or difficulty falling asleep as well as waking up frequently. An even more common problem is frequently waking up even though you don't remember doing so the next day, which interrupts your "deep" sleep. Also, other sleep disorders, such as restless leg syndrome and sleep apnea, may be associated with fibromyalgia.

People with fibromyalgia talk about waking up day after day feeling exhausted with no energy. Usually, people who suffer from fibromyalgia feel more tired in the morning and many go back to sleep during the day to attempt to help their fatigue. Also, it's common for people with fibromyalgia to have great difficulty focusing during the day, a symptom made worse by the fibro fog a lot of them already suffer from. While fibro fog is often attributed to sleep deprivation, it is my belief that fibro fog is not caused by insomnia, but rather made worse by it. The involvement of the cranial nerves, as discussed earlier, is a much likelier culprit.

What do I base my opinion on? I have had dozens of fibromyalgia patients, after being tested with the Neurological Relief Center Technique (NRCT, chapter 5), sit up on my table and report feeling clear as a bell with all their senses restored, regardless of being every bit as sleepy as they first were walking into my office. Sometimes, it is the first time in decades that they feel this fog lift. It is my opinion that the malfunction of the nervous system is directly responsible for this annoying symptom, and that it can be alleviated immediately (although temporarily at first) once the nerve communication is restored.

While almost every patient under allopathic care is prescribed some form of sleep medication, these medications only treat the symptom of sleeplessness, and often poorly. If you want to restore deep sleep, it is crucial that the malfunctioning autonomic nervous system be balanced. Remember, your parasympathetic nervous system is not working correctly, and the parasympathetic nervous system controls your rest. To make matters worse, a study found that the less you sleep, the more you hurt, which, in turn, leads to even poorer sleep.[32]

AVOID BLUE LIGHTS
(AND WE AREN'T TALKING ABOUT THE POLICE)

The color, determined by the wavelength, of the light we see sets our biological clocks, also known as circadian rhythms. In the natural environment, in cavemen (and women) days, this worked out pretty well. During the day, we see all the visible wavelengths provided by the sun: blue, violet, green, yellow, orange, and red light. This light communicates to our bodies that it's daytime, time to shake a tail feather and be active. During this time, secretion of your "sleepy hormone," melatonin, is decreased.

At night, melatonin is not affected by traditionally visible light, which consists of longer wavelengths—the yellows, oranges, and reds that we create through campfires or candles. Melatonin is released by your body like the sandman dishing out dreamtime sand. This allows us to get sleepy right when we are supposed to, together with a large part of the animal kingdom. Lullaby and goodnight.

However, we don't use candles and fire at night anymore. We stare at our TV screens, which emanate blue light. We work on our laptops (as I am doing now)—more blue light. We use our iPhones and other smartphones—you guessed it, blue light. If we wake up in the middle of the night, we can't resist checking our email or our Facebook accounts (maybe somebody else is awake and liked our latest clever status update!)

Ditto iPads and e-readers. (If you are reading this at night on one of those devices, you are suppressing your melatonin as we speak. Finish this paragraph and step away from the blue light.) Our bodies associate blue light with daytime. Blue light wakes up your brain, resets your body clock, and suppresses melatonin all at the same time. The closer your face is to the device, the worse the problem.

If you own an iPad, its blue light emissions can be reduced by adjusting the brightness and switching to white on black mode at night through the "settings" feature. If not, you can now purchase blue light filters for your computer, e-reader, iPad, or smartphone. (Just Google "blue light filters.")

EXHAUSTION

While most people who suffer from fibromyalgia attribute their daily exhaustion to sleeplessness or poor quality sleep, it is usually not the only reason they feel exhausted every day. Adrenal fatigue is also a likely culprit.

Each smaller than a walnut, your two adrenal glands sit on top of your kidneys. These relatively small hormone-producing glands are powerhouses, manufacturing and secreting almost fifty different hormones including adrenalin, cortisol (stress hormone that affects things like fat storage, blood sugar, and blood pressure), estrogen, testosterone, and aldosterone (regulating salt and water levels in the body). They significantly affect the function of every organ and tissue down to every cell in your body.

When these glands are not working properly, your immune system as well as your energy level will be affected. Even your mood may be affected, causing you to see the world through a rather gray lens. When these glands are malfunctioning, your health may also be severely compromised, and you will live below your optimal potential. The adrenal glands are responsible for ensuring that your body's reactions to stress are appropriate to optimize survival, without harming the body in return. For example, the adrenal glands are responsible for secreting protective hormones to help minimize allergic reactions such as swelling.

Adrenal fatigue is a syndrome where these glands malfunction or become fatigued due to working harder and longer than they were designed to do. This may happen after chronic or acute infections, after periods of intense stress such as losing a loved one, or during prolonged stress such as having a stressful job. It may also be caused by malfunctioning of the autonomic nervous system (as is the case in patients who suffer from fibromyalgia). When the brain is "stuck" on sympathetic (fight or flight) overdrive, it is like your body is functioning while you are flooring the gas pedal 24/7. In response, these glands are frantically responding to this unseen stressful situation, for example, by pumping out adrenalin. Eventually, they become exhausted, leading to adrenal fatigue.

So, why don't allopathic doctors generally diagnose adrenal fatigue? Doctors are only taught to look for extreme adrenal malfunction in medical school. This includes Cushing's syndrome, which stems from too much cortisol production, or Addison's disease, which occurs when the adrenal glands don't produce enough cortisol. Traditionally, allopathic physicians check adrenal function by testing ACTH levels, using a bell curve to recognize abnormal levels. The ACTH test (also called the cosyntropin test, tetracosactide test, or Synacthen test) is a test usually ordered and interpreted by endocrinologists to assess the functioning of the adrenal glands by measuring their stress response to adrenocorticotropic (ACTH) hormone.

The problem with this test is that when it is interpreted, only the top and bottom 2 percent of the curve are considered abnormal, yet symptoms of adrenal malfunction occur after 15 percent of the mean on both sides of the curve. In other words, your adrenal glands can be functioning 20 percent below the mean and the rest of your body experiencing all the symptoms of adrenal fatigue, yet most mainstream physicians won't diagnose you with an adrenal problem.

SIGNS OF ADRENAL FATIGUE

- Chronic fatigue and exhaustion (not relieved by sleep), usually worse in the morning and slightly better after 6:00 p.m.

- Decreased sex drive

- Inability to lose weight

- Tendency to carry excess weight in the belly area

- Recurrent infections and decreased immune system

- Lung problems such as bronchitis and asthma

- Allergies

- Sudden dizziness when you stand up from a lying or sitting position

- Muscle aches and weakness

- Depression, sadness, and a general gloomy outlook on life

- Salt or sugar cravings

- Swelling

- Excessive urination

- Hemorrhoids

- Feeling overwhelmed by even minor stress

- Struggling to get through the day

- Symptoms of hypoglycemia (shakiness, dizziness, sweating)

Please note that this list is not meant to replace a professional diagnosis, and that it is not all-inclusive.

HOW TO GET TESTED FOR
ADRENAL FATIGUE AT HOME

In his book *Adrenal Fatigue*, which I highly recommend, James L. Wilson, DC, ND, PhD, describes three methods you may use at home to help determine high probability of adrenal fatigue.

1. **The Iris Contraction Test**
   For this test, you will need a mirror, a stopwatch (or a watch with a second hand), and a darkened room.
   In a darkened room, sit in a chair in front of a mirror. Holding the flashlight at the side of your head, shine it across one eye (not into the eye). Watch what happens to your eye in the mirror. The

pupil should immediately contract when exposed to the light, and stay contracted. If you suffer from adrenal fatigue, however, the pupil won't be able to hold its contraction and will dilate. This dilation will take place within two minutes and last for about thirty to forty-five seconds before it contracts again. Time how long the dilation lasts and record it along with the date. Retest monthly as it serves as an indicator of recovery.

2. **The Blood Pressure Test** (Also known as Ragland's test)
    In order to perform this test, you will need a blood pressure cuff (the type that does not require a stethoscope).
    Make sure you are well hydrated before doing this test; otherwise it will give you a false positive. Lie down quietly for about ten minutes, and then take your blood pressure while still lying down. Then stand up and measure your blood pressure immediately upon standing. Normally blood pressure will rise ten to twenty mmHg from standing up. If your blood pressure drops, you likely have adrenal fatigue. The more severe the drop is, the more severe the adrenal fatigue you are suffering from.

3. **Sergeant's White Line**
    This is the simplest of the home tests. With the capped end of a ballpoint pen, lightly stroke the skin on your abdomen, making a mark about six inches long. Within a few seconds, a line should appear. In a normal reaction, the mark is initially white, but reddens within a few seconds. If you have adrenal fatigue, the line will stay white for about two minutes and will also widen. Please note that if positive, this is an absolute confirmation. However, this test is only present in 40% of people with adrenal fatigue.

ANOTHER TEST WE RECOMMEND:

Saliva testing

Cortisol output by your adrenal glands is one of the most reliable indi-cators of your adrenal function and how well your body is dealing with stress. According to adrenalfatigue.org the cortisol/DHEAS saliva test measures the levels of the stress hormones DHEAS and cortisol in your saliva, and provides an evaluation of how these levels differ throughout the day.

(For more about this test, go to www.adrenalfatigue.org.) Another condition that shares close symptoms with adrenal fatigue is an under-active thyroid gland, or hypothyroidism.

UNDERACTIVE THYROID

(or why looking at a cookie makes you gain two pounds)

The thyroid gland is located in the front of the neck, just below the Adam's apple. The two-inch gland consists of two lobes and is one of the largest endocrine glands in our bodies.

The function of the thyroid gland is to take iodine, found in many foods, such as seaweed, and convert it into thyroid hormones triio-dothyronine (T3) and thyroxine (T4). Thyroid cells are the only cells in the body that can absorb iodine. These cells combine iodine and the amino acid tyrosine to make T3 and T4. T3 and T4 are then released into the bloodstream (the great transportation system) and are cir-culated throughout the body, where they control your metabolism. Metabolism is the conversion of oxygen and calories into energy. This is why the thyroid is known as the fat-burning gland. Every cell in the body depends upon thyroid hormones for regulation of its metabo-lism. In addition, the thyroid gland plays an important role in regulat-ing your body's calcium levels.

The thyroid gland, in turn, is controlled by the hypothalamus (a small area above the brain stem) and the pituitary gland (a gland the size of a peanut, lying beneath the hypothalamus). The hypothalamus helps to coordinate the nervous and endocrine systems. It passes signals to the pituitary gland, which in turn helps to regulate growth, maturation, and metabolism.

When the body is in fight or flight mode, or the autonomic nervous system is activated, the hypothalamus sends signals to the pituitary to secrete several hormones. **Adrenocorticotropic hormone** acts on the adrenal gland to secrete **cortisol,** and TSH **(thyroid-stimulating hormone)** acts on the thyroid gland to secrete **thyroid hormones.**

Remember: the nervous system of a fibromyalgia sufferer is often stuck in sympathetic overdrive.

The result of this response is that the thyroid gland of the patient who suffers from fibromyalgia often stops working correctly. In addition, the patient's immune system is often malfunctioning, leading to auto-immune conditions where the body attacks the thyroid gland.

SIGNS OF A THYROID THAT ISN'T WORKING:

- Fatigue

- Infertility

- Increased sensitivity to cold or heat

- Coarse, dry, scaly, or thick skin

- Constipation

- Difficulty concentrating

- Unexplained weight gain

- Carpal tunnel syndrome

- Puffiness and swelling around the eyes and face

- Hoarseness

- Muscle weakness

- Elevated blood cholesterol level

- Muscle aches, tenderness, and stiffness

- Pain, stiffness, or swelling in your joints

- Heavier than normal or irregular menstrual periods

- Thinning hair

- Slowed heart rate

- Depression

- Impaired memory

- Frequent urination

- Impotence

- Brittle nails

- Poor exercise tolerance

- Panic attacks

- Anxiety

HOW TO GET TESTED FOR A SLUGGISH THYROID

Have both T3 and T4 tested

It is very common for fibromyalgia patients to exhibit many of the symptoms listed above, and test negative for hypothyroidism (sluggish thyroid) when their blood is tested by their allopathic doctor. It doesn't seem to matter if you are exhibiting all of the classic signs of hypothyroidism; if the test indicates that your thyroid is normal, your doctor will typically agree with it. It is up to you, the patient (and the person who cares about your body and health the most), to inform yourself about your symptoms, the tests available to you, the tests needed in your case, and the reasons you ought to have these tests.

TSH:

The old guard's way

The TSH (thyroid stimulating hormone) has become the "gold standard" of thyroid function. When most doctors do a thyroid test, they measure your TSH and decide, based on the test result, whether you have a thyroid problem or not. The typical reference ranges (the numbers below and above which the tests are considered abnormal) are too broad to catch minor fluctuations of the thyroid that may still be symptomatic. Also, these tests are, of course, generalized and do not consider individual differences in physiology.

Even if doctors go a step further, beyond just testing the TSH, and look at your free T4, they will typically not look at your T3 levels. This way, there is no way of knowing if your body is properly converting the T4 it makes into T3. (T4 is the inactive form of thyroid hormone. It must be converted to T3 before the body can use it). This conversion can be decreased because of inflammation or high cortisol levels. Often, regardless of your TSH testing normal, your T3 will be low, resulting in symptoms.

The TSH does not reflect the whole body, but only the function of your brain tissue. According to an expert in the treatment of the thyroid gland, David M. Derry, MD, PhD, thyroid metabolism is controlled locally in the tissue by each organ in very individual and distinct ways. The brain has one mechanism for controlling the amount of thyroid available to the brain, but it is different from that used for other tissues such as the liver. There are many mechanisms by which each tissue controls the amount of thyroid hormone it needs. When TSH is tested, that only reflects thyroid metabolism in *one* of your organs: the brain.

Additionally, monitoring only the TSH levels of someone undergoing treatment for a sluggish thyroid is also going to possibly lead to under-treating the patient. The pituitary cells are the most sensitive cells in the body when it comes to circulating thyroid hormone. Therefore, if your doctor treats hypothyroidism by following the TSH and trying to make it normal, the pituitary cells are happy, but the rest of the body may not be getting nearly the amount it needs. (For more information, please research the work of Dr. Derry.)

Thyroid Antibody Test

If you suffer from fibromyalgia, you should ask your doctor to include the thyroid antibodies tests to detect autoimmune disease, due to the fact that the immune system of a fibromyalgia patient is usually not functioning optimally and autoimmune conditions in this group are common.

Reverse T3

(also known as triiodothyronine)

When your thyroid is healthy, it produces several hormones. These include T1, T2, T3, T4, and RT3 (reverse T3). T4 is a storage hormone that converts into a more active hormone, T3, as needed. Sometimes, the body just needs to get rid of excess T4, and it then converts T4 into RT3. This is mostly done by the liver. Roughly 40 percent of T4 is converted into T3 and 20 percent into RT3. However, if your body is stressed, which results in high cortisol and low adrenals, the conversion into RT3 is sped up to convert about 50 percent of T4 into RT3. This results in low T3 levels, which, as you probably can guess, are not good. Therefore, we suggest that you also get tested for RT3 (reverse T3), especially if your other thyroid tests are inconclusive.

The Temperature Test

It is well known that a slow metabolism is a very common sign of sluggish thyroid glands. Your metabolism will directly affect your body temperature. Therefore, taking your temperature may be an important clue if you suspect that your thyroid gland is underactive.

However, please note that this test is somewhat controversial in its accuracy and should not be used as a standalone diagnostic tool.

The temperature of an adult with a healthy thyroid and a healthy metabolism is (on average) 37.0 degrees Celsius or 98.6 degrees Fahrenheit. The best time to measure this is around 3:00 p.m. If you take your midafternoon temp and find it in the low 98s or even in the 97s, you have been given a strong clue that you may have an underactive thyroid.

Another good time to take your temperature is in the morning before you get out of bed. A normal morning basal temp should be between 97.8 and 98.2. If it's higher, you may be hyperthyroid, and if it's lower, it is possible that you have a sluggish thyroid. You may use the armpit temperature for ten minutes, but taking your oral temperature is just as effective. Be sure to add 1/2 degree to your oral temperature when comparing to the values above.

IS YOUR THYROID SLOW OR YOUR ADRENALS LOW?

(Or both?)

If you suffer from fibromyalgia, it can be very difficult to tell whether you have tired adrenal glands or a slow thyroid gland. Telling the two apart can be a tricky business indeed. To further complicate matters, one will affect the other, and therefore, you may suffer from *both*. If you suspect either of these conditions, you really should get tested for both. However, I want to mention some of the most common symptoms more unique to each condition.

Tired Adrenals	Low Thyroid
Weight gain around the belly area	Generalized weight gain
Temperature fluctuates	Temperature fairly steady
Hair fine and sparse	Hair coarse and sparse
Nails thin and brittle	Nails normal or thick
Sunken eyes	Skin around eyes puffy
Skin dry	Skin oily or moist
Full eyebrows	Sparse eyebrows outer 1/3–1/4
Retains fluids	Fluid retention normal
Ragland's blood pressure test positive	Ragland's test negative
Trembling	No trembling
"Smoothed out" fingerprints	Normal fingerprints

Please note that this list is merely meant to serve as a guide. It is not all-inclusive and should not serve as a definitive diagnostic tool.

ALL THE OTHER SYMPTOMS

If I were to link the autonomic nervous system to each symptom, it would fill an entire book. If you are still skeptical of this fact and you took the time to do even a minimum amount of research, you will find that by using simple tools, such as Google and Google Scholar, you will be able to link the autonomic nervous system directly or indirectly to every major symptom the average fibromyalgia patient suffers from.

One of these symptoms is anxiety, a natural by-product of one's nervous system being convinced that one's survival is being threatened 24/7 (fight-or-flight). Also included is every symptom related to the gut and digestive system, caused by many different factors including inflammation, and its major housekeeper and captain, the parasympathetic nervous system, not being able to do its job, and depression, caused by endocrine abnormalities and sympathetic nervous system dominance (as backed up by studies[33, 34]), to name just a few.

In chapter 9, we will discuss proper supplementation to address some of your most bothersome symptoms and your whole body's health and well-being.

THE SUPPLEMENT MAZE: WHAT IS REALLY NEEDED, AND WHAT REALLY WORKS?

> *The doctor of the future will give no medicine but will interest the patient in the care of the human frame, in diet, and in the cause and prevention of disease.*
> —*Thomas Edison*

> *All those vitamins aren't to keep death at bay, they're to keep deterioration at bay.*
> —*Jeanne Moreau*

F ew things are as confusing as knowing which supplements to take every day. If you are like most fibro patients, you have probably spent a fortune on supplements and natural potions. Most well-meaning people, if they know that you are not well, will bring the newest gimmicky supplement to your attention. Ditto if you sell the special newest multi-marketing you-can-only-pick-these-in-the-Andes-after-four-days-on-the-back-of-a-donkey mountain berry juice. People who don't feel well are easy targets. Sure, the fact that you have only heard about this on late-night infomercials made you suspicious, but you were hurting and desperate, and it wouldn't hurt to try, right?

The problem is, it hurts your pocket, and sometimes all you are doing is adding expensive supplements to your urine. They may pass right through you unabsorbed, they may not benefit you, and they may even harm you. Additionally, people get tired of trying things that don't work, and eventually, they give up. This may keep the patient from finding something that *could* work. I call it "hope fatigue". Eventually you are too tired to even hope, and you give up. This is a dangerous place to be.

Allopathic doctors are generally not very well versed when it comes to vitamins, minerals, or supplements. Up until very recently, recommending vitamins was still frowned upon by the AMA as nonscientific, unconventional, or a form of quackery. Medical schools still do not teach much about diet or supplementation.

> In medical school I had not received any significant instruction on the subject. I was not alone. Only approximately 6 percent of the graduating physicians in the United States have any training in nutrition. Medical students may take elective courses on the topic, but few actually do...the education of most physicians is disease-oriented with a heavy emphasis on pharmaceuticals—we learn about drugs and why and when to use them.
> —Ray D. Strand, MD, the author of Death by Prescription

Scientific studies on supplements and vitamins are hard to find, and you won't find many medical journals publishing papers about natural vitamins and supplements. The reason for this is that a decent study is very, very expensive and some entity, corporation, or interest group usually has to have a financial incentive to pay for these studies. Vitamins are not patentable, so drug companies can't just sell a vitamin the way it appears in nature. In order to be patented so that they won't lose all the millions of dollars they have invested in it, it has to be altered somehow, or made unique.

I have noticed a trend on the Internet: if someone speaks out about something that works, the collective response from other people suffering from the same condition is "show us the research." Even natural or alternative health care providers may greatly disagree when it comes to what is or isn't needed, or what is or isn't good. When I set out on my quest to learn how to help people who suffer from chronic pain, I was especially daunted by supplementation. Just when you think you are comfortable in this field, a new study comes out, contradicting something you were certain was right before.

When I set out to learn how to add nutrition and supplements to my treatment regimen, I didn't have time to reinvent the wheel. I had to find the best and learn from them. When I chose my teachers, I looked at some of the same criteria that I think patients should examine when picking a doctor. How healthy do they appear themselves? Smart doctors follow their own advice. If someone's regime works, it should show in their figure, their skin, and their general vitality. Also, what are their verifiable patient outcomes? Do their patients actually respond to their care?

Based on all the collective knowledge I have gathered over the years from these teachers and nutritional industry experts, I have narrowed my list of vitamins down to the most beneficial and essential. Below is a list of some of the supplements and vitamins that I believe may be helpful to those who suffer from fibromyalgia. Please note that this is not a complete list, as such a list would need a book of its own. Also, this is meant as a guide only, and not meant to replace the advice of your doctor.

Occasionally, you will notice that I recommend a *specific* vitamin or supplement. When I do so, it is merely because I am familiar and satisfied with that supplement's

performance. Rest assured that I am receiving absolutely no financial reward for promoting specific supplements.

THE BASICS:

What every person needs, every single day

All diseases or conditions, from cancer to fibromyalgia, have the following in common: a body with an acidic pH; oxidation of the body; inflammation of the body; and a body that is tired, overloaded, and breaking down. Since we are surrounded by toxins and often overloading out body with chemicals, as discussed in chapter 6, it is most important that we arm our body on a daily basis, optimizing it and making it strong in order to handle any stress we throw at it, be it physical, chemical, or emotional.

Whole Food Multivitamin

It is my opinion that you should take more than the recommended dose (with the exception of iron and a few fat-soluble vitamins listed below), preferably a few in the morning and a few with lunch or dinner. Do not exceed the recommended dose of iron for the day, which is 10 mg for males and 10–15 mg for females. Also, watch out for exceeding the maximum daily recommended intake for Vitamin A (10,000 IU) and Vitamin E (1,500 IU).

Even if you are a healthy eater, it is very difficult to get all the vitamins your body needs today just from your food and beverages. When it comes to a multivitamin, you must choose quality and be prepared to pay a bit more in order to obtain that quality. If you buy your vitamins in a big chain supermarket or pharmacy, chances are that they won't be of superior quality. The companies that manufacture discount vitamins usually use cheap synthetic isolates (incomplete vitamins) combined with chemicals. Your body only absorbs parts of these vitamins, and what is absorbed can't really be used.

According to Joseph Mercola, DO (www.mercola.com), any multivitamin that promises that one a day will be enough is usually a giant waste of money. Even though technology is amazing today, it is still impossible to compress all the vitamins and minerals your body needs into one tiny pill.

Please make sure that any multivitamin you take contains fewer than 100 mcg (that is *micrograms*, not macro!) of copper. Why is this so crucial? Copper has been linked to dementia. A six-year study of more than three thousand seven hundred people sixty-five or older showed that those who consumed at least 1600 micrograms of copper a day added almost *twenty years* to their ages in terms of mental decline.[35]

I recommend Dr. Mercola's **Multivitamin Plus®** (www.mercola.com). He also carries a children's vitamin, but my favorite multivitamin for children is by Natural Vitality: **Kid's Natural Calm Multi Liquid®** (www.naturalvitalitykids.com, or call 866-416-9216).

Vitamin D3

Most people with fibromyalgia are Vitamin D3 deficient. According to Dr. Mercola, "It's important to regularly measure your vitamin D levels to make sure you're maintaining therapeutic levels of 50–70 ng/mL year-round. There are two vitamin D tests: 1,25(OH)D and 25(OH)D. The correct test is 25(OH)D, also called 25-hydroxyvitamin D. This is the better marker of overall D status, and is most strongly associated with overall health." If you live in the United States, Dr. Mercola recommends that you use either tests done by Lab Corp, or the blood spot test that Grassrootshealth.net uses.

In the summer, you may need 2000–5000 IU, or 5000–8000 IU if you do not spend much time in the sun. In the winter, you may need up to 10000 IU. If you are depleted, you may need anywhere from 10000 to 20000 IU for six months to catch up. You will find that this is well above commonly recommended daily vitamin D3 intake. If you are taking these high quantities of vitamin D3, it is vital that you also take vitamin K2. Usually, studies that dispute higher recommended daily intake of vitamin D3 ignore the role of vitamin K2, greatly affecting the outcome of those studies and essentially invalidating them. More on this little-known vitamin will follow shortly.

When your body is exposed to UVB radiation from the sun, it forms Vitamin D3, an oil-soluble steroid hormone. However, in today's world, where we do not spend much time outside and wear sunblock when we do go outside, and where winter months can rob us from sunshine, most people are vitamin D3 deficient. Vitamin D3 is also found in animal organs and fat, cod liver oil, fish, soymilk, and eggs. It is equivalent to the vitamin D3 your body makes when it's exposed to sunshine. You should stay away from the synthetic D2, as it has been shown to be highly toxic at the higher dosages.

Vitamin D3 is absolutely critical for overall good health and disease prevention. It is a major player in cancer prevention. It also positively affects the immune system, auto-immune conditions, insulin, bone density, blood pressure, genetic material, and almost all your organs. Actually, it would probably be easier to list the things vitamin D3 doesn't do than its benefits, since they are so numerous and widespread. A groundbreaking report suggests that taking vitamin D3 supplements may even reduce overall mortality rates: an in-depth analysis of multiple studies found that taking even modest levels of vitamin D supplements was associated with a statistically significant 7 percent reduction in mortality from any cause.[36] Simply put, vitamin

D3 will apparently help you live longer. To me, that is enough motiva-tion to take it.

Vitamin K2 (your calcium taxi)

Adults typically need about 800–1000 micrograms of this vitamin per day. Most people with fibromyalgia are vitamin K2 deficient.

Vitamin K is actually a group of three fat-soluble vitamins. The two main ones are K1 and K2; the third is K3. Chances are you have only heard of vitamin K1, which is found in green leafy vegetables such as kale, broccoli, and spinach, and is very easy to get through your diet. K2 is harder to get and is found in butter, fermented foods like sau-erkraut, and animal products such as goose liver, ground beef, and chicken. (This lack of distinction has created a lot of confusion, and it's one of the reasons why vitamin K2 has been neglected for so long). Vitamin K2 is also produced by bacteria in the colon that convert vita-min K1 into vitamin K2.

K2 prevents cancer (such as liver, prostate, and non-Hodgkin's lymphoma), helps to keep your arteries unblocked, and also works like a taxi for calcium, since it helps to move the calcium where your body needs it most, like your bones and your teeth. Actually, because of that function, you could say that this little-known vitamin is the missing link in fighting osteoporosis. One recent study found that vitamin K2 reduces fractures due to osteoporosis up to a whopping 87 percent.[37]

Because of this, it is crucial that if you are supplementing with vitamin D3 or getting lots of sunshine, you also take vitamin K2. Failure to do so may lead to calcification (for example, of your arteries) due to inappropriate calcium deposits.

Glutathione

*The amount of glutathione you should take
depends upon the form in which you take it.
Please follow manufacturer's recommendation
unless otherwise instructed by your doctor.*

If supplements are boxers, think of glutathione as Rocky Balboa. Glutathione is a tripeptide (a substance that forms when three amino acids link together in a specific order). It is the most powerful antioxidant in your body's arsenal against cancer and toxicity.

Glutathione is a unique antioxidant, since it works *within* the cell rather than from the outside. It maximizes all your other antioxidants, such as vitamin C. As you may be aware, antioxidants eliminate toxins and free radicals from your body. They are also one of your main defense systems against cancer. Glutathione protects the mitochondria in cells against oxidation.

Mitochondria: The cell's powerhouse, producing energy used to fuel the functions of a cell. Think of them as putting gas in your car.

Oxidation: The collective burden placed on cells by the constant production of free radicals in the normal course of metabolism plus whatever other toxins you are exposing your body to on a daily basis.

(While we will address your mitochondria in the next chapter, please be aware for now that the mitochondria in the cells of a patient with fibromyalgia face major challenges and must be supported and repaired as part of a comprehensive fibromyalgia treatment program.)

Glutathione strengthens your immune system, protects you from aging, and plays a major role in DNA repair. Glutathione deficiency has been linked to cancer, Alzheimer's, and many other conditions. Glutathione has also been found to be woefully deficient in people who suffer from fibromyalgia.[38]

Unfortunately, it is very difficult for your body to absorb gluta-thione from your digestive system into your blood. For this reason, please beware of buying oral glutathione supplements, as they are most likely a waste of your money, (bar a few exceptions, like a prod-uct we use fighting cellular inflammation, called Innovita Intracell). Glutathione IVs are effective but not practical for everyone, although certainly worth it. Glutathione suppositories are the next best thing (although granted, nobody's favorite route of delivery). Only about 20 percent of it is absorbed through the skin. According to Dr. Mercola, "The overall top food for maximizing your glutathione is high-quality **whey protein**. It must be cold-pressed whey protein derived from grass-fed cows, and free of hormones, chemicals, and sugar. Quality whey provides all the key amino acids for glutathione production (cys-teine, glycine, and glutamate) and contains a unique cysteine residue (glutamylcysteine) that is highly bioactive in its affinity for converting to glutathione."

Another way you can boost glutathione is by taking the building blocks that make glutathione, thereby boosting your glutathione pro-duction. These include:

N-Acetyl Cysteine

About 500mg a day. If you drink whey, try to take the NAC with your whey.

NAC is a slightly modified version of the sulfur-containing amino acid cysteine. When taken internally, NAC replenishes intracellular levels of the natural antioxidant glutathione. NAC boosts the immune sys-tem, protects against the flu, fights oxidation, decreases inflamma-tion, fights the bad bacteria *Helicobacter pylori*, which cause stomach ulcers, and is responsible for a host of other benefits.

Alpha Lipoic Acid

About 1200mg a day

A fatty acid and a very powerful antioxidant, it destroys free radicals like nobody's business, can function in fat as well as water, and is the only known antioxidant that can get into the brain past the blood-brain barrier. Alpha lipoic acid also has been shown to restore intercellular glutathione. It also fights type II diabetes, helps lupus and erectile dysfunction, detoxifies heavy metals, and much more. It is found in yams, organ meats (particularly red meat), spinach, broccoli, potatoes, yeast, tomatoes, carrots, and beets, to name a few.

Fish Oil

Take two thousand mg a day. Make sure that the oil is heavy-metal and pollution free. I prefer the brands Nordic and Arctic. Do not buy at a chain store. When it comes to fish oil, most oils are contaminated, and, unfortunately, with this supplement you get what you pay for.

Unless you have been living under a rock, you have probably heard by now that fish oil contains omega-3 fatty acid and that is good for you. However, a lot of people still can't tell their omega-3s from their omega-6s. Unfortunately, in modern society, we have become very scared of fats and oils. This has many ill effects on our health. (Remember, eating healthy fat will not make you fat. In fact, it will help you to maintain a healthy weight.)

Omega-3 and omega-6 are both essential fatty acids, meaning we cannot make them on our own and have to get them from our diet. In modern diets, there are few sources of omega-3 fatty acids, mainly the fat of cold-water fish such as sardines, salmon, herring, mackerel, and a few others. They are also found in krill (a small shrimp-like crustacean, the delicacy of whales), and in grass-fed beef. Omega-3s play an important role in lowering inflammation (also in joints), and fighting cancer, depression, and weight gain. They also improve the health of your heart, bones, arteries, brain, and all cells, to name but a few benefits.

In the typical modern diet, omega-6s are everywhere. Although found in seeds and nuts, they are also found in refined vegetable oils, fast food, soy, junk food, snack food, cookies, and sweets. If it's the type of food you scarf down and feel guilty after, you can bet your bottom dollar that it contains omega-6s. Ideally, the omega-6/omega-3 ratio should be 1:1, although 2:1 or 3:1 is still acceptable. Unfortunately, a lot of people consume these fats in a ratio of 20:1 or even 50:1! This is why you must up your omega-3s and cut down on your omega-6s.

Now, I know this is not riveting stuff, but bear with me. There are two omega-3 fatty acids that our bodies *must* have: DHA (or docosahexaenoic acid), and EPA (eicosapentaenoic acid). Plant sources contain a precursor omega-3 (alpha-linolenic acid, called ALA) that the body must convert to EPA and DHA. EPA and DHA are the building blocks for hormones that control immune function, blood clotting, and cell growth as well as components of cell membranes. They are found in, for example, garbanzo beans (the beans that that delicious stuff called hummus is made from), as well as nuts such as walnuts and flaxseeds.

Take 100mg of flaxseed oil daily.

Pomegranate Juice

Take 8 oz daily

This is one of the only juices we advocate drinking. In general, juice contains massive amounts of sugar (even natural) that spikes your blood glucose levels and leads to cellular inflammation. Although pomegranate juice is not really a supplement, research from around the world confirms that pomegranate is one of nature's most concentrated sources of antioxidants. Pomegranate juice protects your heart, lowers blood pressure, fights cancer and aging, and most astoundingly, according to one new study, can reverse atherosclerosis,[39] something that used to be believed not to be possible.

FIBRO SPECIFIC SUPPLEMENTS

Adrenal Support

(Please refer to chapter 9 to understand why you need adrenal support) We recommend 'High Absorption Stress & Adrenal Support' chewable tablets by New Health Products (1-800-828-1108), one tablet three times a day.

Supplements designed specifically for adrenal fatigue will nourish, strengthen, support, and optimize your adrenal function. They will also help to support homeostatic balance in the body and optimize biochemical communication in order to obtain a healthy response by these glands to stress. All eight B vitamins are essential for healthy adrenal function, as they act as catalysts in adrenal functions. Of the eight, the most important are **vitamins B3 (niacin), B5 (pantothenic acid)**, and **B6 (pyridoxine). B vitamins should be taken sublingually (dissolved in the mouth). The reason for this is that it** delivers B12 directly to the bloodstream, bypassing the digestive system, which results in its maximum absorption.

Magnesium, Your "Stress Mineral"

> *We recommended Natural Calm™ by Natural Vitality™, available on Amazon.com (dosage as recommended by manufacturer unless directed otherwise by your health care professional).*

Involved in pain perception pathways and muscle contraction, magnesium may improve tenderness and pain. It is also involved in healthy brain and neurological function and bone density. Magnesium is beneficial in helping your body cope with stress and in helping you sleep. Enough said.

Selenomethionine

> *Selenomethionine is a form of selenium. I recommend taking 55 mcg of selenomethionine per day. Selenomethionine has the best bioavailability with an absorption rate of roughly 90 percent. It is organic and yeast-free. When compared with other selenium supplements, selenomethionine proves to be the most applicable and safest for long-term therapeutic use.*

Selenium is a trace element that is naturally present in many foods such as Brazil nuts (up to seventy micrograms per nut!), liver, shellfish, and sunflower seeds, to name but a few. It is also available as a dietary supplement. Selenium is required by the body for proper functioning of the thyroid gland, for glutathione production, and for mercury detoxification. It may help protect against free radical damage, cancer, and autoimmune disease. A deficiency in selenium can lead to pain in the muscles and joints, unhealthy hair, and white spots on the fingernails. Selenium deficiency has been linked to fibromyalgia: in one trial, symptoms improved in 95 percent of patients supplemented with selenium for at least four weeks.[40]

Ubiquinol (or Coenzyme Q10)

If you're over forty, Dr. Mercola highly recommends taking a reduced form of coenzyme Q10 called ubiquinol, because it's far more effectively absorbed by your body. (Ubiquinol is the reduced, electron-rich form of coenzyme Q10).

If you take statin (high cholesterol) drugs, it is crucial to take coenzyme Q10, since statin drugs interfere with your body's natural CoQ10 production.

Take 150 mg twice a day for two weeks, and after that, 100 mg a day for the rest of your life.

Coenzyme Q10 is almost like a vitamin, but since the body naturally makes it, it isn't called a vitamin. CoQ10 (as it is also commonly known) has been called "the single most crucial nutrient to supplement every cell in your body" by Dr. Mercola. Your cells use it to produce energy your body needs for cell growth and maintenance. Coenzymes help enzymes work to digest food and perform other body processes, and they help protect the heart and skeletal muscles.

Coenzyme Q10 also functions as an antioxidant that protects the body from damage caused by harmful molecules. CoQ10 has been shown to help prevent or retard development of a fatty liver related to obesity, to fight inflammation, free radical damage and cancer, to protect against high blood pressure, and to help prevent heart attacks.

Last but not least, and sure to appeal to everybody's vanity, CoQ10 is an excellent tool in your anti-aging arsenal. Think of this supplement as your fairy godmother, giving you a makeover from the inside out. One study in Japan found a *significant* slowing down of the aging process in a group of mice that were given Ubiquinol.[41] In addition, clinical trials have consistently shown that CoQ10 reduces fibromyalgia symptoms such as pain and fatigue.[42, 43]

CoQ10 is naturally present in small amounts in a wide variety of foods, but levels are particularly high in organ meats such as <u>heart</u>, <u>liver</u>, and <u>kidney</u>, as well as beef, sardines, mackerel, and peanuts.

L-Carnitine

Although most people do not need extra L-carnitine, people who suffer from fibromyalgia may benefit from supplementation. Vegetarians may also need to supplement. Best taken in its activated form, Acetyl-l-carnitine.

Take 250–500mg a day as needed for muscle pain.

L-carnitine is an amino acid that is directly involved in cellular fatty acid metabolism. Although it can be obtained from your diet (red meats are a particularly rich source), it is also produced in your liver and kidneys. Most of the carnitine in your body is stored in your muscles and heart, where it is needed to transfer fatty acids into mitochondria so they can be oxidized for energy. An L-carnitine deficiency may cause muscle pain due to inefficient cellular energy metabolism (mitochondrial myopathy), common in fibromyalgia.[44] L-carnitine has also been shown to improve mental clarity and overall energy, and to fight aging, type II diabetes, and cancer.

D-Ribose

500 mg three times a day for four weeks and 500 mg twice a day after as needed.

This may be the most important supplement in your fibromyalgia and chronic fatigue arsenal. D-ribose is a naturally occurring sugar that has been shown to support the production and recycling of ATP (think of it as fuel for your car), which helps to increase energy production in stressed tissues. It may even be effective to alleviate migraines.

One study found that when D-ribose was given to fibromyalgia sufferers it resulted in a significant improvement in energy, sleep, mental clarity, pain intensity, and overall well-being. Approximately 66 percent of fibromyalgia patients experienced significant improvement while on D-ribose during this study.[45]

Malic Acid

Most effective when combined with magnesium.

Start at a daily recommended dosage of 600 mg twice a day, coupled with 150 mg of magnesium twice per day, and slowly increase your levels to 1200 mg of malic acid twice per day coupled with 300 milligrams of magnesium, also twice per day, over 2–3 months.

Malic acid is an organic acid made by all living organisms. It is also responsible for that pleasantly sour tang in apples and other fruits, and is sometimes referred to as "fruit acid." Malic acid is involved in energy production in muscle cells. It is necessary for glucose metabolism, which is important for nourishing muscles and nerves. Malic acid increases ATP production (cellular fuel). It will enhance your mood and may help reduce muscle discomfort and overall pain in those who suffer from fibromyalgia. One study found a significant decrease in pain in patients suffering from fibromyalgia and supplementing with malic acid.[46]

Curcumin

Take 300 mg a day. Contraindicated for those on blood-thinning medications or those with gall bladder disease.

Curcumin is the key component of turmeric, and is responsible for the spice's distinctive mustard-yellow color. This spice is popular in the Far East, especially in curry-spice blends. It's a member of the ginger family and comes from a root just like ginger. Curcumin is a proven antioxidant and a powerful anti-inflammatory. Some research shows it can even boost your immunity, may show benefits in fighting cancer, and is a powerful antiviral. It has also shown benefits in helping to relieve the symptoms of irritable bowel syndrome (IBS) as well as arthritis and menstrual cramps. It also positively affects pain associated with fibromyalgia.[47]

Zinc

22 mg twice per day. Taking zinc together with vitamin C may cause nausea.

Zinc is an essential mineral that is naturally present in some foods such as oysters, crabs, wheat germ, pumpkin seeds, watermelon seeds, roast beef, dark chocolate and cocoa powder, lamb, and peanuts. Low blood levels of zinc are associated with the number of tender points in fibromyalgia patients.[48] Yet another study found that serum levels of those patients with chronic fatigue syndrome were significantly lower.[49]

In addition, zinc is required by your body for maintaining a sense of smell, keeping a healthy immune system, building proteins, triggering enzymes, tissue growth and repair, skin health, and making DNA. Zinc also helps the cells in your body communicate by functioning as a neurotransmitter. A deficiency in zinc can lead to stunted growth, diarrhea, impotence, hair loss, stretch marks, eye and skin lesions, impaired appetite, and depressed immunity. In addition, taking extra zinc during pregnancy has been shown to be much more effective at preventing stretch marks than rubbing oil or lotion on your tummy.

Please note that *too* much zinc may cause nausea, vomiting, and diarrhea. If you experience these side effects, please back off your dosage.

CHAPTER 10

CONDITIONS THAT MAY RESEMBLE OR OVERLAP WITH FIBROMYALGIA

And after all, what is a lie? It is but
the truth in a masquerade.
—Lord Byron

I think it's a very valuable thing for a doctor to learn how to
do research, to learn how to approach research, something
there isn't time to teach them in medical school. They don't
really learn how to approach a problem, and yet diagnosis
is a problem; and I think that year spent in research is
extremely valuable to them.
—Gertrude B. Elion

Fibromyalgia is a tricky beast. It is often mistaken for other conditions and, just as if that doesn't make it complicated enough, it often coexists *with* other conditions, making it especially nightmarish in the sense that it is very complicated and difficult to diagnose. After working with fibromyalgia for so long, a doctor will usually become familiar with the conditions mistaken for (or coexisting with) fibromyalgia. Interestingly enough, I have noticed that patients with these conditions usually respond very well to the same treatment I use for fibromyalgia. A common cause would explain the similarities between these conditions, and would also explain why a somewhat similar treatment plan should prove successful in treating them, despite their obvious differences.

RSD/CRPS

(Reflex Sympathetic Dystrophy/Chronic Regional Pain Syndrome)

Of all the conditions I treat, I am probably most passionate about RSD/CRPS. Of the most painful conditions known to man, this one has to top out as the most painful one on the chronic pain scale. It most often will start in a limb, after a seemingly not too uncommon injury or invasion to the body of some sort. (Think fracture, bunion surgery, ankle sprain, knee surgery, or even an injury to the nail.) Instead of the injury recovering, patients report that their pain intensifies at an alarming rate.

Patients new to my office with this condition will often report their pain to be as high as one hundred on the ten scale, and it is largely untouched by pain medications such as opiates. While no specific statistics are available, it is not, in my experience, uncommon for patients suffering from RSD/CRPS to consider suicide...not because they don't want to live, but because they don't want to hurt anymore.

The most common symptom of RSD is chronic pain, frequently described by patients as burning or stinging. We are not talking mild pain either, but more that of the blowtorch variety, all the time. Patients also suffer from extreme skin sensitivity, so that even clothing, the brush of a sheet, or the wind on their skin is unbearable. The humidity may make it worse. Ditto sunshine, cold, or hot temperatures.

Other symptoms include swelling, profuse sweating, nail changes, skin rashes (frequently mistaken for fungus or allergies), and color and temperature abnormalities at or near the injury site. Patients may also experience muscle spasms, weakness, tremors, extreme fatigue, problems sleeping, frequent infections, cardiac complications, digestive problems, fever, headaches, migraines, spinal problems, and severe pain when eating. The hallmarks of this disease are sweating, color changes, temperature changes, and cold sensitivity. This may lead to the limb contracting and to bone loss, easily identifiable by a bone scan.

In some people, the disease is confined to the affected area, but in as many as 70 percent of patients it spreads to adjacent parts of the body or crosses over to affect the same area of the opposite limb. It may also spread to areas unrelated to the injury, such as the trunk, internal organs, optic nerves, and scalp.

I consider this condition terrifying and rather creepy. Why? There is the obvious and constant threat of the RSD spreading. These patients live in fear of needing surgery or injuring another body part, which could cause that to happen. Even an innocent needle prick can cause a whole new symptom site to develop.

In addition, these patients are *set up* to develop RSD/CRPS before they get injured, but they don't know it. They are walking around like a ticking time bomb, innocently undergoing, for instance, foot or knee surgery, all along not knowing that this "perfect storm" is waiting to stir inside of them, unleashing its terrifying pain and suffering.

Although it's not known exactly how many people have RSD worldwide, it is estimated that as many as eight million suffer from the disease in the United States alone, and that it complicates as many as 5 percent of all injuries. Typical age of onset is the midthirties, yet children and the elderly also develop the disorder. Just like fibromyalgia, it affects women more often than men.

Dr. Robert DeMartino (who contributed to this book), always tells his patients that the "S" in RSD stands for sympathetic. It is remarkable how this whole part of the autonomic nervous system is neglected in the treatment of that condition. Remember how the sympathetic nervous system (chapter 7) plays an important role in the development of fibromyalgia? This is also the case in RSD/CRPS, in our opinion most often caused by an old upper cervical injury (like a whiplash injury) that may or may not be coupled with spinal stenosis.

As a matter of fact, we treat the neurological symptoms of RSD/CRPS much the same as fibromyalgia, with marked success. The involvement of the sympathetic nervous system also explains the cardiac and digestive problems that RSD/CRPS patients often develop. Remember, when the sympathetic nervous system is stuck on "on," the heart is racing, and the parasympathetic nervous system running digestion is MIA.

People who suffer from RSD/CRPS will often develop fibromyalgia, and people who already suffer from fibromyalgia may be at a higher risk than the normal population to develop RSD/CRPS. For this reason, it is important to be familiar with the signs and symptoms of RSD/CRPS, as treatment within the first three months is crucial and it is difficult for doctors to diagnose. Current conventional treatment includes ketamine infusions (ketamine is a horse tranquilizer) or ketamine-induced comas, which have the same effect on the nervous system as hitting CTL, ALT, and DEL together on your keyboard to reboot your computer (this treatment is not FDA-approved and only available in Mexico and Germany), spinal cord stimulators, some rehabilitation, and pain management.

In our clinics we balance and correct the autonomic dysfunction, thereby normalizing the sympathetic nervous system, coupled with other treatments like frequency-specific microcurrent (more about that to follow later).

RSD/CRPS pain will usually start in one limb, where it is more widespread in fibromyalgia, although it is not unusual for fibromyalgia to only be symptomatic on one side of the body. Think of the pain from fibromyalgia as that of a deep bruise and RSD/CRPS as a severe burn or the feeling that you get when you scrape the skin off of your knees. People with fibromyalgia also usually suffer more intense fatigue, although this is not a golden rule.

BRENDA'S STORY

(RSD/CRPS Patient)

My name is Brenda Wood; I am forty-six years old and married, with three children, three grandchildren, and twin grandbabies on the way. Yay! How exciting. My story started with me having a heel spur removed from my right foot in December of 2009. Two weeks after the surgery I was able to remove my boot, but after the very first step I took, I knew something was not right. I was in more pain than before the surgery. How could this be? The doctor told me to give it some time and come back in two weeks. Two weeks passed and the pain was worse. I had sharp, shooting pain, swelling, and burning in my right foot; my foot was always cold and always hurt. I went back, in more pain than before the surgery. My doctor didn't know what the problem could be.

After weeks of going back and forth I went to another doctor, and thus my two-year journey began, going to doctor after doctor after doctor. I had one put me in a cast just to see if it would help because he just didn't know what to do. I became so frustrated, not being able to work, not being able to do the things I used to do; even little things seemed so hard to do. By now I was on long-term disability and I was thinking, "What will happen if I can never go back to work? I won't be able to help my husband financially." I didn't know what to do!

Finally, I went to see a neurologist, who listened to my story and checked the medical records I had brought from all the doctors I had seen. He went out of the office, came back in, looked at my foot, and said "I believe you have chronic pain syndrome or reflex sympathetic dystrophy (RSD)." He then told me it's a neurological condition with the nerves over-firing. I felt a lump in my throat and tears welling up in my eyes. I was just so thankful that some-one had finally found out what was wrong. After two years, I had finally been diagnosed. Even though he did tell me there was not much they could do for this and I would have it the rest of my life, I was just so thankful to finally have a name for whatever was wrong. I felt like no one believed me; I had people ask me, "How are you doing today? You look good, you're walking around—you must be OK."

The one person who always seemed to understand and believe me was my husband, who, by the way, has been incredible through all this. Not everyone is as lucky as I am with their spouse believing them about the pain. I have met so many people with this disease and still their families don't believe them. People think, because they can't see anything wrong with you, that there is nothing wrong. RSD is a monster of a disease. It robs you of your life. It makes you think you're crazy.

After being diagnosed with RSD, I began to see a pain management doctor. He started me on lots of medications, none of which worked. I went and had nerve blocks every week for about three to four months. They were a waste of time and money. I had to drive about two hours every week to have this done and it just was not helping. I went to my next appointment with my pain management doctor and told them that the nerve blocks and medications did not help. He said, "We can try you on the stimulator that they insert into your back." As soon as they said that, I wanted to run. I knew I was not letting anyone cut into me again. Surgery was what started my RSD and I was not having anyone cut into me. I had read that once you have RSD it could spread, especially to a new surgery site. I had to figure something out, and fast.

I had been on Facebook one day and saw an ad for a teleconference for RSD. I mentioned it to my husband and we decided to sign up to listen. This doctor was saying she could possibly tell within the first ten minutes of the treatment if she would be able to help me, which I thought was too good to be true. Really? Ten minutes? I thought this sounded too good to be true. But what did I have to lose? If I went there and it didn't help, I'd leave. Just gas money spent. If I did get relief, I would consider staying for treatment.

My husband and I talked it over for a little while, thinking that if I didn't go I could be missing out on getting relief and getting my life back. We decided I was going. I called and talked to the doctor's assistant. She was so friendly and she set us up with an appointment. We drove to Fayetteville, Arkansas from Springville, Tennessee.

When we walked into her office, we were surprised by how friendly everyone was. Dr. Katinka talked privately with my husband and myself, and then ordered X-rays and a test to see where my problem spots were. I then came back later that afternoon and was called to Dr. Katinka's table. She started to tell me what she would be doing, and explained every step. She had asked what pain level I was at and I had told her about an eight; then she started the treatment and was able to get me down to about a two. I started to feel less pain, less burning. This is not possible, I thought. Was this my imagination?

I stayed at the hotel for a month, receiving treatments everyday. After a month I was to go home for a month, and then return for another month of treatments. After about three weeks at home, the pain started up again. Pat, my husband, called Dr. Katinka and told her what was going on. She said I needed to get back there as soon as possible. The longer I was gone, the harder it would be to get the pain under control. We left shortly after that and I began another month of treatment.

I can remember that one time, when Pat came to visit me, I was walking after a treatment and the ladies in the office said he had become emotional because I was walking without pain. I was walking! I hadn't done that much before the treatments. During treatment I began to take myself off my medications, as I wanted to be sure they were not masking anything. I had to know if the treatments were really working. I was eating healthier and noticed I was losing weight. I was able to do more walking than I was in the past without pain.

I could not believe how I was feeling. I felt like I was getting my life back. It was amazing. I had begun to miss my family dearly and wanted to go home. I was about done with my month and was getting excited to see everyone. I missed my home with my husband, my children, and my grandchildren. It was time for me to leave after my second month. I knew I would miss Dr. Katinka and her amazing staff. They are more like friends now. I had met so many wonderful people who were patients and became friends; we shared a bond because of our chronic pain.

Dr. Katinka is an amazing person, an amazing doctor. I am so grateful to her for everything she has done for me. She has given me my life back. I wish that every RSD patient could see her. I wish they too could feel as good as I do. Yes, there are days I get pain and burning, but it always calms down. It is nothing like it was before. Here I am writing this today and having a pain-free day. Thank you, Dr. Katinka.

CHRONIC FATIGUE SYNDROME

As you may guess, the name of this syndrome says it all. When you suffer from this you are chronically, debilitatingly tired, and no readily apparent underlying medical cause can be found. Sleep becomes an obsession, but in a cruel twist, does not relieve your fatigue. This syndrome is usually only considered to be an "official" diagnosis once you have been fatigued for six consecutive months or more.

CFS patients may also suffer from headaches, a weakened immune system, depression, increased sensitivity to light, sounds, and smells, digestive issues, and possible cardiac problems (all of which symptoms are also found in those who suffer from fibromyalgia). Physical or mental stress may make this syndrome worse. Patients who suffer from this should have both their adrenal and thyroid function thoroughly tested as described in chapter 8.

Once again, it is my belief that an unbalanced autonomic nervous system is responsible for the majority of cases of chronic fatigue syndrome, as the parasympathetic (resting and digesting) system is turned off and the sympathetic (fight or flight) systems are "on" all the time. Adrenal support and supplementation are crucial for these patients, as is balancing the autonomic nervous system so that the parasympathetic nervous system is turned back on.

Fibromyalgia is closely related to chronic fatigue syndrome. In an article published in Fibromyalgia AWARE in 2002, a publication of the National Fibromyalgia Association, Charles W. Lapp, MD, an expert and researcher in chronic fatigue syndrome as well as fibromyalgia, stated that "about 70 percent of persons with CFS meet criteria for FM and about 70 percent of persons with FM also meet criteria for CFS." However, please note that not every patient with fibromyalgia has chronic fatigue, and vice versa.

There are some differences between fibromyalgia and chronic fatigue syndrome. For instance, Substance P (a neurotransmitter that transmits pain signals) is elevated in FM but not CFS.

RNaseL (a cellular antiviral enzyme), a specific biomarker whose presence indicates that the body put up a vigorous fight against some kind of viral attack, is frequently elevated in CFS but not in FM and is now used to test for CFS. However, please note that this biomarker may also be elevated in multiple sclerosis.

Often CFS will be triggered by a flu-like or infectious illness, while FM is more often triggered by some kind of trauma to the body (e.g. a car accident).

LUPUS ERYTHEMATOSUS

Lupus is a chronic inflammatory disease that is actually a collection of autoimmune conditions. These conditions develop when the immune system mistakenly attacks normal, healthy organs, affecting entire body systems. Some of the organs that may be affected include the skin, joints, blood cells, heart, kidneys, and lungs. Lupus affects up to ten times as many women as men. Lupus is more common among African Americans and Asians. Most patients will have times when the disease is active followed by times when the disease is inactive, also referred to as remission.

Lupus may manifest as a systemic disease, or systemic lupus erythematosus (SLE), the most common and most dangerous form. It may also present in a purely cutaneous form known as incomplete lupus erythematosus. Lupus has four main types: neonatal, drug-induced, discoid, and systemic. Lupus may be further divided into further subcategories too complicated to discuss here.

The symptoms of lupus vary from person to person. The most distinctive symptom (and sign) of lupus, a facial rash that resembles the wings of a butterfly across both cheeks, occurs in many but not all cases of lupus. Other symptoms may include swelling, arthritis in the joints, fever, fatigue, weight loss, blood clots, hair loss in spots or around the hairline, mouth sores, indigestion, nausea, stomach pain, heartburn, heart problems, kidney problems, and poor circulation to the fingers and toes. Pregnant women may have miscarriages.

Lupus is treated traditionally with a multi-disciplinary approach, including medications and immune suppression, which may be uniquely tailored based on the patient's symptoms. In our clinics, we have noticed that the neurological symptoms of lupus respond very well once the autonomic nervous system is balanced. These patients also need massive supplementation, rebuilding of the gut, and immune support. Sadly, lupus only has a 68 percent twenty-year survival rate, and may be very serious in the long term.

Fibromyalgia is often mistaken for lupus and vice versa. Lupus patients will typically not exhibit the same tender points that patients with fibromyalgia do. Lupus patients also will often have the butterfly rash made worse by the sun and visible arthritis in their joints.

Lupus will most often show a positive antinuclear antibody (ANA) test (although this test is not failure-proof), or show certain antibodies pointing to a faulty immune system, called anti-double-strand DNA (anti-dsDNA), anti-Smith (referred to as anti-Sm), or antiphospholipid antibodies. They may also show a false positive blood test for syphilis (meaning they do not really have this infection but appear to.)

MULTIPLE SCLEROSIS

Multiple sclerosis (MS) is a chronic, often disabling disease that was previously thought to be caused when the body's immune system attacks its own central nervous system (CNS), resulting in the myelin sheaths (think of them as insulation) around nerve cells in parts of the brain and spinal cord being damaged, in turn leading to loss of myelin and scarring. These changes affect the ability of nerve cells to communicate, resulting in a wide range of signs and symptoms. These symptoms may be mild, such as numbness in the limbs, or severe, such as loss of vision or paralysis.

The progress, severity, and specific symptoms of MS are some-what unpredictable and may vary from one person to another. Typical symptoms may include fatigue, loss of vision/hearing, double vision or visual blurriness in the central visual field that affects only one eye, weakness of the arms or legs, neuropathy (tingling, pain or numbness) in the limbs, speech impairment, difficulty balancing, and bowel or bladder incontinence.

A diagnosis is often made after a careful history and neurological exam (the skills of the neurologist are crucial here), a spinal tap, blood tests (to rule out conditions with similar symptoms), MRI (to show lesions), and a neurological test called an evoked potential test (to show nerve damage).

The model for immune system dysfunction leaves one obvious question unanswered: *why* does the immune system turn on itself in the first place? After all, this seems to be a common occurrence in multiple conditions including MS, fibromyalgia, lupus, and rheumatoid arthritis. All share an immune system gone haywire and now on the prowl, damaging its own body. Since the immune system is governed by the central nervous system, it would make sense that there might be a link between this system and the immune system's nutty behavior.

A groundbreaking study performed in 2011 using upright MRIs found: *"Multiple sclerosis may be bio-mechanical in origin wherein traumatic injuries to the cervical spine result in cervical pathologies that impede the normal circulation of CSF to and from the brain."*[50] In layman's terms, this means that multiple sclerosis may also be caused by injuries to the cervical spine, such as car accidents. While more studies are needed, we find this research eye-opening and very promising indeed. In our work, we have noticed great changes in the neurological symptoms of MS when the upper cervical spine was treated and corrected.

Although the symptoms of fibromyalgia and MS have marked differences, we do find that these conditions may sometimes (especially early on) be misdiagnosed as each other. The tests mentioned above should be able to accurately distinguish MS from fibromyalgia.

Please keep in mind that, especially in a case where someone suffered from past upper cervical trauma, both conditions may exist in one patient.

LYME DISEASE

If you have Lyme disease, or know someone with Lyme disease, hang on to your chair, as we are about to give you a whole new look at this disease.

The most accepted and universal belief is that Lyme disease (Lyme Borreliosis) is an infectious tick-borne disease caused by at least three species of bacteria belonging to the genus Borrelia. Early symptoms may include fever, fatigue, headaches, or depression. A characteristic circular skin rash called erythema migrans (EM) appears around the bite. Left untreated, later symptoms may involve the heart, joints, and central nervous system. In most cases, the symptoms are eliminated by antibiotics, if treated early. However, delayed or inadequate treatment can lead to more serious symptoms, which may be disabling and difficult to treat.

Lyme disease is divided into three stages. First is early localized infection, where the infection has not yet spread throughout the entire body. During this stage, roughly 80 percent of patients will develop the characteristic "bulls-eye" rash at the site of the bite. The second stage is the early disseminated infection, when the infection spreads through the bloodstream within days to weeks after the onset of the initial local infection. This happens in only one in three hundred to four hundred cases, where again only 10 to 15 percent of patients may subsequently develop neurological symptoms such as meningitis (an infection of the membranes around the brain and spinal cord), shooting pains, and palsy of the face (where the muscles in the face become paralyzed).

Late disseminated infection (stage III) may occur after several months, when a small percentage of patients (about 5 percent) go on to develop severe and chronic symptoms that affect many parts of the body. This may include the brain, nerves, eyes, joints, and heart. Other serious symptoms may include "frank" psychosis, arthritis, vertigo, and bladder problems.

The current theory about Lyme Borreliosis was formulated in 1977. At that time, Allen C. Steere, MD, and his colleagues, who were studying rheumatology at Yale University (he is now a professor at Harvard), discovered a "new disease" called Lyme Borreliosis after substantial prospective trials. In 1983, the first international conference on Lyme disease took place at Yale University. However, in 2012, Dr. Steere stated that long-term symptoms seen in Lyme disease were, in his opinion, caused more by an immune system failure rather than an infection, and would not benefit from antibiotics.

The problem with the current Lyme disease theory is that not all people bitten by an infected tick become sick with Lyme disease. Therefore, it stands to reason that the immunity of the host must have something to do with it, and all the problems can't be caused by bacteria alone (we come full circle, once again back to the immune system). It follows then that part of a well-rounded treatment program should be to strengthen the body and immune system from the inside.

Treatment steps for lyme disease

It is our opinion that unless the infection is less than two weeks old, it should not be treated with antibiotics. Please find a health care practitioner knowledgeable in Lyme disease who can guide you through the following treatment steps:

4) Get tested for heavy metal toxicity.

5) Detoxify your body of all toxins.

6) Improve the overall health of your body with diet, supplementation, and specific treatments aimed toward improving the immune system.

Lab testing will rule in or rule out Lyme disease in most cases.

Tests include the Borrelia-DNA via PCR (polymerase chain reaction), which may be used to diagnose an acute infection in the first few weeks, but has proven to be rather inaccurate after that. If a suspected infection is older, an enzyme-linked immunoassay (ELISA) test to look for IgG and IgM antibodies (which may give false negatives early on) or a Western blot test may be used.

DIGESTIVE DISORDERS SUCH AS IBS (IRRITABLE BOWEL SYNDROME), DIVERTICULITIS, CELIAC DISEASE, CROHN'S DISEASE AND GLUTEN INTOLERANCE

Think of your gut not as a system to be broken down into parts and organs that may individually break down, but as a whole system where every part is connected to every other part, affecting your entire health, mood, longevity, and well-being.

Your digestive system is usually treated as separate parts working independently of each other, only to be tested when they malfunction or break down, through laboratory work or scopes. After this extensive testing, you will usually find yourself stamped with a disease name, told to avoid certain foods, given medication, or operated upon. The gut is a dynamic, powerful, intricate system, where the health of every part affects the health of every other part as well as the health and immunity of the entire body that it nourishes.

One of the main areas of the body that do not communicate with the nervous system in the autonomic dysfunction seen in most cases of fibromyalgia is the digestive system. Remember, the digestive system is controlled by the parasympathetic (or resting and digesting) nervous system. Think of the parasympathetic nervous system as the housekeeper or captain. Any miscommunication between this area and the nervous system will eventually lead to a multitude of problems, like yeast overgrowth, an imbalance in good bacteria, indigestion, malabsorption of nutrients, and possible damage of structures.

While we think of our intestines as merely a factory where nutrients are extracted from food and waste expelled from our bodies, there is so much more to them. It is a little-known fact that most of the body's serotonin (at least 90 percent) is synthesized and stored in the intestines. We even have a "second brain" in our intestines. Known as the enteric nervous system, the second brain consists of neurons embedded in the walls of our gut, which measures about thirty feet (or nine meters) end to end from the esophagus to the anus. Know how you get "butterflies in your stomach"? It is connected to that nervous system. We actually *do* feel emotions in our guts.

The health of the gut is very closely linked to the health of the nervous system. Just like the larger brain in the head, researchers say, this system sends and receives impulses, records experiences, and responds to emotions. Its nerve cells are bathed in and influenced by the same neurotransmitters. The gut can upset the brain just as the brain can upset the gut.

DEPRESSION AND YOUR GUT

When your gut becomes damaged or inflamed, whether from emotional stress, candida, or toxins, undigested food particles and toxins enter your bloodstream through openings in your damaged gut (also called a leaky gut), where they are attacked by your immune system, resulting in the release of cytokines and inflammation in different parts of your body and brain. Cytokines are small proteins used as messengers by the immune system and are released in response to inflammation or inflammatory conditions. Cytokines have a powerful effect on brain chemistry and function and have been linked to depression and brain fog.

The following may cause digestive symptoms (especially in patients suffering from fibromyalgia):

- Autonomic (parasympathetic) nervous system dysfunction, turning "off" digestion and the immune system in the gut

- Overuse of antibiotics causing an imbalance in good vs. bad bacteria

- Candida overgrowth resulting from a weakened immune system, heavy metal toxicity, or not enough good bacteria in the gut

- A poor diet low in fiber, acidic in nature, and high in sugar and saturated fats

- Medications adversely affecting the gut

- Weakened digestive enzymes, resulting in food not being completely digested

- Food sensitivities or allergies

The health of your digestive system is directly linked to the health of your immune system. Almost 70 percent of the immune system resides in your intestinal tract.[51] This branch of the immune system, made up of billions of friendly bacteria and yeast, is responsible for many functions including proper nutrient absorption, production of vital nutrients (produced by the bacteria in your gut), detoxification and alkalization of the body, and last but not least, one of the main weapons your body uses in fighting against bad bacteria.

While we do not have the luxury of space to discuss every digestive problem or diagnosis in detail, we feel strongly that the digestive system of every patient suffering from fibromyalgia must be treated as if it is not well.

The Basic Steps Necessary To Heal The Digestive System:

1) Detoxify

2) Change your diet (please refer to chapter 11)

3) Rebuild (please refer to chapter 13 or www.tamethefibro-beast.com)

4) Nourish the body with healthy and proper vitamins, minerals and supplements (please refer to chapter 9)

Every patient who suffers from fibromyalgia should rebuild and restore their digestive system.

INTERSTITIAL CYSTITIS

Interstitial cystitis (IC) or painful bladder syndrome (PBS) is a chronic inflammation of the bladder wall that causes nagging pain and severe discomfort. Symptoms often include a sense of urgency and increased frequency of urination. While a healthy adult urinates on average about six times a day, a person with IC may urinate up to seventy times in twenty-four hours, including several times at night, interrupting their sleep.

Inflammation associated with IC causes the lining to scar and the bladder to become stiff and less elastic, which may affect the way the bladder can expand. In about 90 percent of IC cases, there are pinpoint spots of bleeding visible in the lining. In up to 10 percent of cases, ulcers known as Hunner's patches may form on the bladder wall. As if this condition isn't uncomfortable enough, it may also worsen during menstruation and can cause intercourse to be painful for both sexes.

A large survey of six thousand seven hundred and eighty-three patients with IC/PBS found that 40 percent of patients with IC also suffered from allergies, while 30 percent suffered from irritable bowel syndrome.

Cranberry extract (not juice) has proven to be somewhat successful, as well as a supplement called D-mannose. D-mannose is a type of sugar that has been shown to relieve IC/PBS. It is theorized that D-mannose might treat the deficiency caused by a genetic defect that causes abnormal breakdown and production of mannose or that D-mannose might prevent certain kinds of bacteria from sticking to the walls of the urinary tract and causing infection. (This supplement can be ordered at mercola.com.)

Interestingly enough, as if following a trail of breadcrumbs, the newest research again points to the autonomic nervous system as a direct cause of IC/PBS, where it is shown that people with IC/PBS also exhibit an overactive sympathetic nervous system.[52]

TEMPOROMANDIBULAR DISORDER (TMD)

TMD (temporomandibular disorder) refers to a group of usually painful conditions that affect the joints of the jaw (temporomandibular joint or TMJ). It may also affect the nerves of the head and face and the associated muscles used in movement of the jaw and neck.

The symptoms of TMD include limited movement or locking of the jaw, clenching or grinding of the teeth (especially at night), a "tired" feeling in the face, limited ability to open the mouth very wide, clicking, popping, or grinding noises in the joints of the jaw, difficulty chewing, a warm or inflamed feeling in the muscles of the jaw, swelling of the face, radiating pain in the face, neck, or shoulders, a sudden, major change in the way the upper and lower teeth fit together, and unexplained headaches or facial pain that may be dull, aching, or constant.

As you may guess, once again, studies have clearly linked autonomic nervous system dysfunction to TMD.[53] Therefore, it is crucial when addressing this disorder that the underlying neurological cause be treated, and not merely the symptoms, whether by biomechanical, chemical, or surgical intervention.

TRIGEMINAL NEURALGIA

Trigeminal neuralgia (also known as tic douloureux) is a nerve disorder that causes sharp, sudden, searing, electric-shock-like facial pains and affects about one out of every fifteen thousand people, although it is much more common among those who also suffer from fibromyalgia. The pain comes from a cranial nerve called the trigeminal nerve and usually affects one side of the lower face and jaw, although symptoms may appear near the eyes, ears, nose, jaw, or lips. Many experts say trigeminal neuralgia is the most unbearably painful human condition, and for this reason, it is tragically also known as "the suicide disease", just like RSD/CRPS, or fibromyalgia in severe cases.

Trigeminal neuralgia has been linked with autonomic nervous system dysfunction.[54] In addition, at least one study has linked it to upper cervical trauma such as whiplash injuries.[55] Medically, this condition is treated with medications or surgery. We believe that this condition must be approached in such a way that the autonomic nervous system dysfunction is balanced and corrected. In addition, we correct any upper cervical misalignment present and rehabilitate the trigeminal nerve in our treatment approach.

RESTLESS LEG SYNDROME

Restless leg syndrome (RLS) is a neurological disorder characterized by unpleasant sensations in the legs (and sometimes other parts of the body such as arms, trunk, or head), and an uncontrollable or overwhelming urge to move them. People with RLS may constantly move their legs (or other affected parts) to minimize or prevent these sensations.

Symptoms may include throbbing or a pulling and crawling sensation occurring primarily at night. Resting or lying down actually worsens these sensations, making it particularly disruptive to sleep and rest. The sensations range in severity from uncomfortable to irritating to painful. RLS is very common and may affect up to 10 percent of the population, especially the fibromyalgia population. Medically, this condition is usually addressed through medications. At least one study has found a definitive link between sympathetic nervous system dysfunction and RLS.[56]

As I said earlier, it is impossible to address each separate condition or symptom associated with fibromyalgia. It is my sincere hope that if you suffer from any of the above symptoms or conditions together with fibromyalgia, you will start to think of the body as a system where every part is connected to every other part, and where the nervous system governs all. If you can spot the patterns between all your symptoms, you can begin to find your way out of the seemingly neverending labyrinth of symptoms full of dead ends and suffering.

It is my hope that the patient of the future will not only be interested in the numbing of every symptom of their disease, syndrome, or condition, but also be interested in the underlying cause of those symptoms and in how to effectively treat them, thereby living a better quality life where overall health and quality of life is the ultimate goal.

CHAPTER 11

EATING FOR YOUR HEALTH: YOUR DIET

---

*Let your food be your medicine and
your medicine your food.*
—Hippocrates

If you keep good food in your fridge, you will eat good food.
—Erick McAdams

I believe that our body is a precious gift, and that we have to be a good steward of it. We have an opportunity to either add to our health or detract from it every time we eat or drink something. After we swallow this food, it is now up to our body to either maximize the healing potential of the food we just ate, or minimize the damage caused by it in the best way it can, until it gets too tired to do so. If you suffer from fibromyalgia, you need the support that good nutritious food can give you even more than the average person and can afford damage from bad food even less.

The problem is, if you are like most people, you are probably as confused as a chameleon in a bag of Skittle candies about what exactly you should or should not eat. As you have so much on your plate, it is my sincere belief that a healthy diet should follow sound principles and be kept simple. Healthy eating should be so simple that you can follow it most days of the rest of your life. Give a man a fish and you feed him for a day; teach a man to fish and you feed him for a lifetime.

With that in mind, we will explain some broad principles, followed by some daily food suggestions and suggestions of things to avoid like a toxic friend.

> *"Keep it simple, stupid."*
> —Kelly Johnson

WHAT IS YOUR PH? ACID VS. ALKALINE

If you ever took even the most basic chemistry class, you probably know that any liquid has either an alkaline or an acid pH. Our bodies were designed to be alkaline by nature (at a tightly controlled pH of 7.4), and acidic by function—meaning that the waste products our cells produce when they work are usually acidic. Your alkalinity is not only determined by your diet but also by the toxins you are exposed to, the air that you breathe, the liquids you drink, how much you exercise, and even your thoughts.

The stability of your blood pH is protected from swings, since even a tiny swing in pH may kill you. In fact, this is a major argument by those who oppose the acid/alkaline principle. According to them, your blood is protected from swings in pH and therefore should not be affected by an acidic diet. While that is true, when it comes to your urine (and the rest of your body), it is a different story. When your diet is very acidic, your urine chemistry is altered in profound ways, possibly resulting in kidney stones, which you may have heard aren't much fun.

When your diet is mostly acidic, it takes a big toll on your body. It will cause cellular inflammation (the last thing you need) and aging and besides the aforementioned kidney stones, may also cause gallstones and osteoporosis, the latter taking place because your body will basically "dissolve" bone in order to buffer the acid.[57] Think of your bones as a bank, and of calcium as money. When your diet is too acidic, your body has to "borrow" calcium from your bones order to buffer it, with every intention of "paying back" this loan once you clean up your act. The problem is, most people never do.

An acidic diet will also decrease the body's ability to repair damaged cells, as well as its ability to absorb minerals and other nutrients. This results in a decrease in the energy production of the cells (already an area of major concern in those who suffer from fibromyalgia), lowering their ability to detoxify heavy metals and other toxins. This may cause cancer cells to thrive and make it more vulnerable to fatigue, general wear and tear, and illness.

On the other hand, your health will greatly improve if your diet is more alkaline. Your skin will look younger (since osteoporosis has been tied to the appearance of wrinkles), your bones will be stronger, and you will be less likely to be overweight. An alkaline diet has even been tied to decreased low back pain[58] (almost a universal complaint of those suffering from fibromyalgia).

It is fairly simple to test your saliva and urine pH at home armed with some pH paper. I recommend that every person with fibromyalgia do it. For a more detailed guide to this testing, you may go here: http://www.energiseforlife.com/wordpress/2006/04/12/alkaline-test-how-to-test-your-ph-levels-saliva-urine/

For a complete list of acid/alkaline foods, you can turn to Google or websites like http://rense.com/1.mpicons/acidalka.htm.

Generally, vegetables and fruits (and most nuts and seeds) are alkaline, and animal products such as meat and cheese, refined carbs, junk food, sugar, and pastas are acidic foods. As a general rule, if you are sick, you should aim for an 80/20 balance, where 80 percent of the food you eat has an alkaline pH or effect on the body (for instance, even though a lemon is acidic, it will have an alkalizing *effect* on your body). Please be advised that your body might be so excited because of this change that it may actually start "spring cleaning" and detoxifying old piled-up toxins.

As discussed earlier in this book, this may not feel too pleasant and can often not be tolerated by those who suffer from fibromyalgia. If this happens—in the form if diarrhea, headaches, or a general unpleasant feeling—back off from the alkaline food and go about it more slowly. You will have to find your own pace. In order to *maintain* health, a 70/30 (70 percent alkaline foods, 30 percent acid foods) daily balance is recommended. A great supplement to alkalize your body on a daily basis is green barley powder.

Remember, it's OK to mess up some of the time, as long as you eat good, mostly alkaline food most of the time. No one is taking away your ice cream forever!

IT'S ALL ABOUT OMEGA-3/OMEGA-6S

Earlier in this book we gave a detailed discussion of the importance of omega-3/omega-6 fatty acid balance in your body (chapter 9, under "Fish Oil"). Just to recap: There are two types of fats essential to your body, omega-3 and omega-6. However, the typical modern human being consumes far too many omega-6 fats in their diet while consuming very low levels of omega-3. The primary sources of omega-6 are soy, corn, grapeseed, canola, safflower and sunflower oils. These oils are used in tons of mass-produced food and fast food and are overabundant in the typical diet, which explains our excess omega-6 levels. Avoid or limit these oils. Omega-3, meanwhile, is typically found in flaxseed, virgin coconut, krill, and fish oils.

By far, the best type of omega-3 fats are those found in that last category, fish. That's because the omega-3 in fish is high in two fatty acids crucial to human health, DHA and EPA. These two fatty acids are pivotal in preventing heart disease, cancer, and many other diseases. Unfortunately, the ocean has become a more contaminated environment, and care must be taken to avoid the intake of heavy metals together with your fish oil. Do not buy cheap fish oil supplements at large stores. For recommended brands, please go to "Fish Oil" in chapter 9.

Remember, the ideal ratio of omega-6 to omega-3 fats is 1:1, a ratio maintained by our ancestors for millions of years. Today, though, according to Dr. Mercola and other sources, our ratio of omega-6 to omega-3 averages anywhere from 20:1 to 50:1! This imbalance may contribute to autoimmune conditions, cancer, pain, Alzheimer's disease, and cellular inflammation (of particular concern for those who suffer from fibromyalgia), to name a few. In your case, it is crucial that you work toward a healthier omega-3/omega-6 balance, since this is one of the main tools in fighting inflammation.

YOUR CELLS ON FIRE: THE ROLE OF CELLULAR INFLAMMATION.

Inflammation is the normal expected immune response of tissues due to any injury. Signs of acute inflammation include heat, pain, swelling, and redness at the site of the injury. Your body may also become stiff in the area (for example, a sprained ankle joint), thereby protecting the joint from excessive movements while it is healing (remember how smart your body is?). This type of acute inflammation is normally a localized, protective, logical response following infection or trauma.

However, if the agent causing the inflammation persists for a prolonged period of time, the inflammation becomes chronic, as in the case of fibromyalgia. People who suffer from autoimmune conditions and allergies are particularly vulnerable to exaggerated inflammatory responses.

Inflammation may be fought through a healthy diet relatively low in protein, (good quality protein), healthy oils and fats, lots of fruits and vegetables, plenty of omega-3s (restoring the balance in the central nervous system) and supplementation. It is also *crucial* to rebuild the gut in order to decrease cellular inflammation (addressed later in this book).

Stay in the range of 40g (for women) to 55g (for men) of animal protein a day (unless you are an Olympic athlete).

(These numbers were obtained by the CDC (Centers for Disease Control). Children's required protein intake may fall anywhere between 13 and 40 grams depending on their age). Note that pregnant women also require higher daily intakes of protein. http://www.cdc.gov/nutrition/everyone/basics/protein.html

At least one study has found that the more protein you eat, the more calcium you lose in your urine.[59] Also, remember that a major goal for those who suffer from fibromyalgia is to cut down on cellular inflammation (see above). Excess protein will cause cellular inflammation.

Good quality protein is far more important than quantity. We recommend healthy whey in smoothies as a great source of protein (go to mercola.com for whey recommendations), or a product called "Dream Protein," available on Amazon.com

"You are what you eat, so don't be fast, easy, cheap, or fake."

- Unknown

ANIMALS ARE WHAT THEY EAT: TRY TO KEEP YOUR ANIMAL PRODUCTS NATURAL.

Study after study has shown that the omega-3/omega-6 balances in grain fed animals such as bison, chicken, and beef are not healthy.[60,61,62]

When you eat beef, make sure that it is grass-fed beef. The longer cattle eat grain, the greater the fatty acid imbalance (omega-3/omega-6) in their meat. After even two hundred days (standard in the United States) it has been shown that omega-6/omega-3 ratios may exceed 20 to 1. Venison is generally better for you than beef, unless the deer was exposed to soy.

Also, make sure that when you eat eggs or chicken or turkey you only consume the eggs or meat of chickens and turkey that eat vegetables high in omega-3 fats, along with insects and grass, supplemented with fruit and very small amounts of corn. According to Dr. Mercola, range-fed eggs have an omega-6 /omega-3 ratio of 1.5 to 1, whereas the egg you typically buy at a supermarket has a ratio of 20 to 1. Please avoid "omega-3 enriched" eggs. While this sounds like a good idea in theory, these chickens are usually not fed in a healthy way.

Farm-raised fish such as tilapia and catfish have been found to be especially detrimental to your health, based on at least one study of its effect on your omega-3/omega-6 ratio.[63] Some people even call tilapia the "bacon of the ocean" because of this. Make sure that, as a rule, the fish you eat is not farm-raised, as the emphasis in the industry is to get these fish produced in mass quantities and to breed them to be as large as possible.

WATCH THOSE CARBS

Few other areas in nutrition have been debated as hotly and passionately as carbohydrates. At least one major Japanese study found that the intelligence and actual anatomy of the brains of schoolchildren were altered based on the amount and type of carbs they consumed in the morning for breakfast.[64] Another study found a direct link between refined carbs and an increased risk of stroke in women.[65]

How healthy or unhealthy a specific carb is usually depends upon its glycemic index (GI), or how fast that specific carb raises your blood sugar after eating it relative to pure glucose (which has a GI of one hundred). Generally, the higher the GI, the worse the food is for you, the faster it raises your insulin, and the more inflammation it causes. While I am not a big believer in completely cutting out an entire food group, I do believe that it will benefit fibromyalgia patients especially to limit their carbohydrate consumption to about two servings of healthy carbohydrates a day.

Carbs are actually the one food group not essential for survival. However, as we said before, we prefer moderation instead of elimination. Your body much prefers getting its carbs from fruits and vegetables, as they have a low GI and release blood sugar slowly. Try to limit your intake of healthy grains (let's call them moderate carbs) to no more than 20 percent of your daily diet. These include all those carbs that you were probably taught were essential for health, including brown and white rice, barley, potatoes, corn, millet, nuts, and whole-grain bread.

Try to eliminate unhealthy carbs (bad carbs) as much as you can, except as a special treat every now and then. I am not telling you to bake a hemp cake for your birthday, but just to be good most of the time. Unhealthy carbs include white bread, bagels, pretzels, and anything looking irresistible at your local bakery (doughnuts, cream puffs, and croissants, for instance), as well as processed cakes and treats like Twinkies (yes, they are coming back) and so on. This group also includes sugar, high fructose corn syrup, and fructose. Please use honey or stevia (a natural sweetener) instead.

As an added bonus, cutting down on your carbs will positively affect your health as well as your weight.

BOTTOMS UP

We have all heard that we need eight eight-ounce glasses of water every day. However, this information is outdated. The Institute of

Medicine set its general guidelines for women to consume a total of ninety-one ounces (about two point seven liters) per day. For men, it's about one hundred and twenty-five ounces a day (or three point seven liters). Keep in mind that those numbers include fluid from all the food and beverages you consume combined. Depending on your diet, about 25 percent of the water you consume comes from your food. The simplest way to tell whether you drink enough water is to look at your urine. It should be light yellow (unless you take vitamins or supplements affecting the color). It should also not have a strong odor.

Hate drinking water? You are not alone. We can actually dampen our desire for water (thirsting mechanism) over time if our bodies get accustomed to constant dehydration. Age can also have this affect. Don't be fooled, however. Every cell in your body needs water.

When it comes to what kind of water to drink, always ask yourself, "What would nature do?" We do not recommend that you drink water straight out of a faucet due to additives and toxicity issues. Ionized water is alkalized by electricity splitting the water molecules, without added minerals. In nature, water flows over rocks and through soil, collecting naturally alkalizing minerals such as calcium and magnesium. If you drink this type of water, be sure to add trace minerals or lemon juice to your water (more about that in a bit). Also, never drink water that is too alkaline (pH above eight), as your body will counter this by acidifying itself.

Avoid bottled water in plastic bottles unless the bottle is BPA-free, as BPA (a harmful chemical found in plastics) often leaches into the water, especially if heated up (never leave bottled water in a hot car). Distilled and reverse osmosis water is "dead" water that will leach minerals from your body. Always add the juice of half a lemon to filtered water, as this will add minerals back into the water and is also naturally alkalizing. (Do rinse your mouth out after with plain water in order to protect your teeth). You may also add trace minerals in liquid form.

IT TAKES MORE THAN ONE APPLE A DAY

Unless you have been living under a rock, you have probably heard that fruits and veggies are good for you. As a general rule, you should try to eat five to seven cups of fruits and vegetables a day. Vegetables and fruits will lower your risk of heart disease, stroke, osteoporosis, certain kinds of cancers, kidney and gallstones, and oxidative stress, and increase your mental clarity.[66,67] They also contain enzymes that assist digestion, and are full of antioxidants and phytochemicals that help to boost your immune system.

Eating your fruits and veggies has also been shown to be very beneficial to those who suffer from chronic conditions (of particular interest to you). As a general rule, vegetables rebuild your cells, and fruits clean (detoxify) them. One study, reviewing two hundred other studies studying the relationship between fruits and vegetables and cancer, found overwhelming evidence that *"Persons with low fruit and vegetable intake (at least the lower one-fourth of the population) experience about twice the risk of cancer compared with those with high intake, even after control for potentially confounding factors"*.[68]

Because most people with chronic diseases are also somewhat insulin resistant, it is best to keep your fruit/vegetable ratio at 30 percent fruit to 70 percent vegetables. A few additional things to remember: raw is always best (keeping the enzymes, nutrients, and alkalinity intact), and for my readers from the South, where nothing is above frying, deep-frying it pretty much turns any vegetable into the equivalent of a doughnut. Also, potatoes aren't vegetables, and, while buying all organic is certainly too expensive for most of us, I really do suggest that you avoid "dirty" fruits and vegetables, since eating them does more harm than good, unless you buy them organic. On the other hand, you may buy "clean" produce anywhere.

- **Dirty fruit**
Peaches, cherries, apples, nectarines, strawberries, grapes (imported), and pears.

- **Clean fruit**

Cantaloupes, grape fruit, kiwi fruit, mangoes, papayas, and pineapples.

- **Dirty vegetables**

Bell peppers, celery, kale, lettuce, carrots, cherry tomatoes, cucumbers, hot peppers, potatoes (technically a starch), spinach, collard greens, and summer squash.

- **Clean vegetables**

Avocadoes, asparagus, cabbage, sweet peas, sweet corn, egg-plant, mushrooms, onions, and sweet potatoes.

Everything not on these lists and not certified organic should be treated with suspicion and peeled or washed when possible. To make your own vegetable wash, combine equal amounts of white vinegar and clean water. Mix and spray onto hard-skinned produce, or soak soft-skinned produce for two minutes in solution in a bowl. Rinse under a faucet.

> Tip: Get into a habit of making one or two smoothies
> every day. This way it is easier to consume larger
> amounts of produce in its raw form and to get the
> needed servings every day. For breakfast, I use a
> Vitamix® blender (worth its weight in gold, although
> any good blender will work), and add one or two fruits
> such as orange, lemon, lime, blueberries, pineapple,
> and apple, and four to five vegetables such as kale,
> spinach, beets, carrots, and even radishes with water,
> whey powder, coconut oil, flax seed oil, fish oil
> (undetected by taste if of superior quality) ice,
> stevia (to sweeten it), cinnamon, and ginger root.
> Experiment with the tastes you like and start
> with more fruits to acclimate to the taste.

FATS DON'T MAKE YOU FAT. LET ME REPEAT THAT.
Fats don't make you fat.

One of the worse rumors that ever got started regarding food is that fat is bad for you and leads to heart attacks, strokes, and will cause you to have a body that is less than svelte. Eating a low-fat diet was believed to be the holy grail of healthful eating and low cholesterol for decades. Seeing a fantastic marketing opportunity, and also giving the public what it wanted, food companies reinvented and re-engineered thousands of foods to be lower in fat or fat-free, often increasing the salt, sugar, or chemicals in these foods to make up for lost flavor.

Fats provide essential fatty acids, which are not made by the body and must be obtained from food. The essential fatty acids (linoleic and linolenic acid) are necessary for many biologic processes in the body, such as vitamin and mineral absorption (why it is good to take vitamin D together with healthy fat or oil), mineral absorption, revving up your metabolism (that's right, weight loss!), brain function, fighting cellular inflammation, heart health, and many more.[67]

When it comes to being bad for you or fattening, it is not the amount of fats that count, but the quality and types. In addition to the 1:1 omega-3/omega-6 balance we already discussed, you also need some other fats. Let's look at an overview of those to eat and those to avoid and the categories these fats are divided into.

Saturated Fats

Some good and some bad, such as butter (limit), ice cream (limit), cream (limit), fatty meats (fine if grass-fed), avocado (good for you), nuts (good for you, with the exception of peanut butter), coconut (good for you *if* of good quality and virgin, and great for cooking, as it is not very damaged by heat. Make sure that it smells like coconuts.)

EATING FOR YOUR HEALTH: YOUR DIET

If you have heard that coconut oil is bad for you, that information is outdated and incorrect, as most old studies on coconut oil used hydrogenated or partially hydrogenated coconut oil.

Unsaturated Fats

Divided into monounsaturated fats (olive and canola oils) and polyunsaturated fats (sunflower, fish, safflower, corn, and soybean oils). Of the above list, we prefer using olive oil (best if not heated above 250°F/121°C) and fish oil.

Hydrogenated and Partially Hydrogenated Fats

Hydrogenation is the chemical process by which liquid saturated oils are turned into solid fat. In other words, these are hardened or partially hardened oils (such as hard butter). Foods containing hydrogenated oils should be avoided because they contain high levels of trans fatty acids, which are linked to heart disease, increased "bad" cholesterol (LDL), and decreased "good" cholesterol (HDL).

Trans Fatty Acids

These fats form when hydrogen atoms are added to an unsaturated fat such as vegetable oil (hydrogenation), and can raise LDL ("bad" cholesterol) and lower HDL levels ("good cholesterol"). Trans fatty acids are found in fried foods, commercial baked goods (donuts, cookies, crackers, chips), processed foods, and margarines.

You get the general idea. Higher omega-3s and lower omega-6s are good, some saturated fats are good and even necessary (contrary to long-held popular belief), most unsaturated fats are good (but shouldn't be heated as a general rule), and hydrogenated, partially hydrogenated, and trans fats should be avoided as diligently as swimsuit models avoid cream puffs.

ALLERGIES AND OTHER IRRITATING FOODS

People who suffer from fibromyalgia almost always suffer from food allergies, resulting from a "confused" immune system and a digestive system not working properly, leaking large particles into the bloodstream, where they are attacked by the immune system as foreign particles. While we are huge proponents of first restoring proper nervous system communication and then rebuilding the digestive systems of those who suffer from fibromyalgia, it is crucial to stop pouring irritating foods into that system.

If there is a specific food that you crave, like sugar, there is a good chance that you are allergic to that food. Isn't that a strange oxymoron? It is theorized that the reason this happens is that when a food allergy causes chemical and physical stress inside your body, your body produces endorphins, which comfort you and make you feel good, thus making you crave more of it. One of my vices is Starbucks coffee. I find myself especially craving it when my energy is low or I am emotionally in a bad spot, just as a treat or a pick-me-up.

Allergies to food will make the whole repair process rather ineffective, like a dog chasing its own tail. Also, it will increase cellular inflammation and therefore pain. First, get a proper blood test to determine which foods you are allergic to. I suggest that you get tested for food-specific reactions to three different antibodies: IgG, IgE, and IgA, which typically result from noticeable reactions to specific foods.

One of the ways your immune system defends against invaders like viruses, bacteria, or a foreign particle, is by producing cells called antibodies, also called immunoglobulins. There are five major immunoglobulins: IgA, IgD, IgE, IgG, and IgM.

Only IgE reactions are considered true food *allergies*, and will require a blood draw. IgE reactions typically occur within minutes of exposure to or ingestion of a specific food. Common IgE reactions include trouble breathing, wheezing, flushing, a feeling of getting hot, hives, itchy watery eyes, swelling, and anxiety.

Food sensitivity is a term that usually refers to delayed immune reactions to foods, or non-immune reactions to food. The symptoms of food sensitivities and allergies are quite different. While a food allergy normally causes an immediate reaction, the symptoms of food sensitivities may not be as obvious as those of food allergies. The reasons for this are that often food sensitivities are delayed, and the reactions are not as clearly identifiable.

The following are just a few examples of symptoms of food sensitivities: fatigue, lethargy, anger, exhaustion (especially after eating), headaches, migraines, mood swings, depression, restlessness, water retention, joint pain, gas, bloating, constipation, diarrhea, and indigestion. IgG and IgA react to foods and can be detected from a dry strip sample of blood.

Eight foods cause 90 percent of all allergies in the USA. These are peanuts, tree nuts (such as walnuts), milk, eggs, wheat, soy, fish, and shellfish.

In addition, people who suffer from fibromyalgia have been shown to be sensitive to nightshade vegetables. Nightshade fruits and vegetables are said to grow "in the shade of the night" (rather creepy, if you ask me), and contain chemicals such as alkaloids that can increase arthritic pain and symptoms. The most common nightshades are potatoes, tomatoes, peppers (sweet and hot), eggplant, tomatillos, pimentos (usually used to stuff olives), cherries, paprika, and cayenne.

Golden rule: Try to eat well 80 percent of the time, and allow yourself to mess up 20 percent of the time. Striving for excellence is more sustainable than striving for perfection.

THE EXCEPTION TO THE 80/20 RULE: THE NO-NO LIST.

Trust me, the following foods are not worth the harm they cause you. They are toxic, nasty, cancer-causing, pain-elevating, hormone-disrupting, and generally wreak havoc upon your body. To make this list, these chemicals and additives had to be particularly offensive to your health and well-being.

The culprits are:

- Artificial sweeteners (as discussed in chapter 4) such as aspartame (NutraSweet, Equal), saccharin (Sweet'N' Low, SugarTwin), and sucralose (Splenda)

- Diet sodas and chewing gum containing these sweeteners

- High fructose corn syrup

- Artificial coloring agents (usually a color followed by a number, such as FD&C Blue No. 1), that has been shown by at least one study to interfere with your body's energy (ATP) production,[68] already a problem area in those with fibromyalgia

- Monosodium glutamate (MSG)

- Major hormone-disrupting **butylatedhydroxyanisole (**BHA) and butylatedhydroxytoluene (BHT)

- Sodium nitrite and sodium nitrate (potentially linked to diabetes and colon cancer)

- Potassium bromate (potentially carcinogenic and illegal in Canada, Europe, China, and Brazil)

- Recombinant bovine growth hormone (rBGH)

- Sodium benzoate and potassium benzoate (benzene is a known carcinogen that is also linked with serious thyroid damage, especially if, for example, soda bottles in plastic containing benzene are exposed to heat in transport)

So remember, don't try to be perfect, be excellent. Stop eating mindlessly and conveniently. Educate yourself so that you can learn how to make healthy choices on your own, and you can be like a strong oak tree, not swayed this way or that by the media every time a new wind of change or nutritional fad blows through. You must arm yourself with basic nutritional knowledge and daily habits that will withstand the test of time, and that will allow you to feed and honor your body with the best kind of medicine there is: healthy, nutritious food.

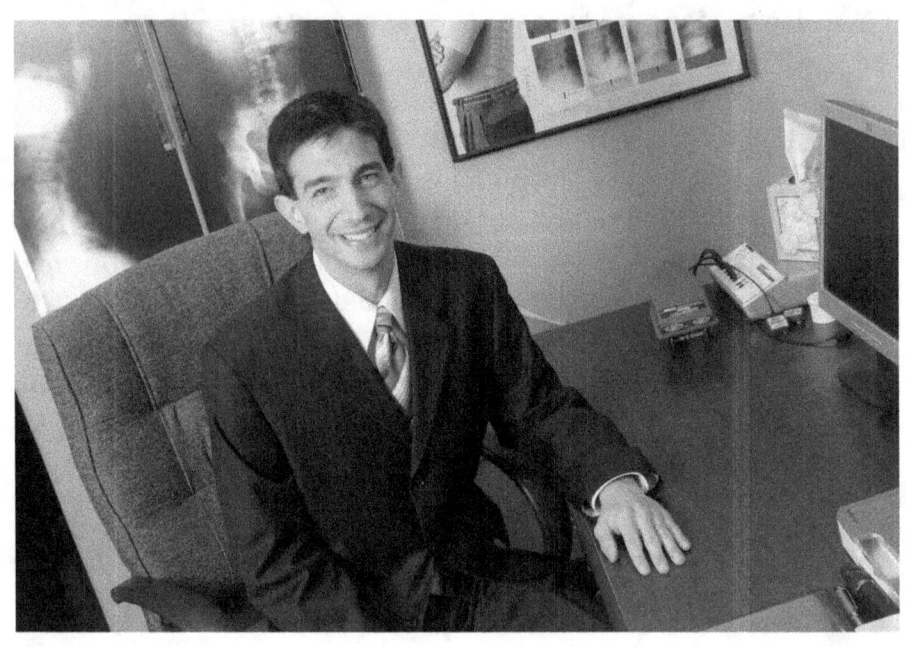

CHAPTER 12

[HEMISTRY GONE WRONG

(BY ROBERT V DEMARTINO, DC, QN)

> *But I think my mistakes became the chemistry for my miracles. I think that my tests became my testimonies.*
> —*T. D. Jakes*
>
> *Why have all the pieces joined together to create such a cruel fate?*
> —*Ichtys*

I t is an honor and privilege to be able to take part in an undertaking of this size, writing a comprehensive "how to" guide when taking on one of the more difficult disease processes known as fibromyalgia. My name is Dr. Rob DeMartino and I have the task of walking you through the science, the reasoning, and the action steps that you must take in order to begin the process of healing. As Dr. Katinka so eloquently stated at the beginning of this book, we are all put on this earth with a specific mission and a purpose. I'd like to share with you a little of my path and how I ended up where I am.

MY STORY

My parents call me the miracle baby. They desperately wanted a second child. My sister, born almost seven years before me, was proof that it could happen. Still, for those seven years my parents tried and tried to no avail. They tried every pill, potion, and lotion known to man. Nothing worked. As many of these stories go, right as they were about to give up hope, it happened for them. Nine months later I arrived and everyone couldn't have been happier.

Six months later, my older sister developed some knee pain. The doctors termed it "normal knee pain." However, it kept hanging around. One doctor would call it growing pains; another suggested that perhaps she was trying to gain attention because a new baby had just arrived. Eventually the doctors settled on a diagnosis of rheumatoid arthritis. This was a curious diagnosis, as the hallmark of RA is that it is uniform and bilateral. That means that if one knee has it, so does the other. But this was only on her one knee. Four years passed, and by the time that they realized it was aggressive bone cancer, it was far too late. She fought and my family fought for her, and I wish my story had a happy ending. How I wish that. Sadly, a few weeks short of her seventeenth birthday, she passed away.

Needless to say, because of this experience, my childhood was a bit atypical. I grew up around hospitals. I grew up around illness. While all the other kids wanted to be firefighters and astronauts, I would profess that I wanted to be an oncologist when I grew up. My destiny was pretty well laid out. My purpose, my mission in this life was to make sure that no one would have to go through what my family did. Not on my watch. However, while my mind was determined, my body failed.

Soon after she passed, I began having debilitating migraine headaches. The light sensitivity, the crushing sensation, the vomiting and praying that when I could finally get to sleep and wake up, it would be gone. My parents, who are extraordinary people, took me all over trying to get me help. After all, we lived in New York, just outside New York City. We had access to the best doctors in the world and I saw them all. Even my sister's cancer doctors took pity on our family and called in favors with their doctor friends to try and help me. It was always the same story. They told me that they could help me and that they would figure it out. I had so many X-rays and MRIs and CAT scans that it is a miracle I didn't glow. All the tests would come back with the same answer: we don't see anything wrong. Sounds like great news, right? But I still had the same headaches. Same problems, no relief. That soon turned to no hope.

I went four years having a migraine every other day. I missed school, I missed spending time with friends, I missed fun, and I was missing out on life. As crazy as it sounds, I thank God for that one day I was feeling well enough that I went out to play basketball and took a pretty nasty fall. My low back was in a lot of pain, and pain ran down both my legs. My parents took me to the chiropractor. To be honest, when I filled out the paperwork, I didn't even put down that I had headaches. It didn't even occur to me to tell him about that. In my mind, I wasn't there for that; I just wanted this back pain gone.

When the chiropractor examined me, he touched my neck and immediately asked if I had neck pain or headaches. I was kind of surprised but went on to explain to him that I had these headaches and had been all over the city and no one could help. Imagine my surprise when he stated that he thought he could help me. I politely said, "Oh, OK. Thanks." To myself I thought, "Yeah, right. Just fix my back, dude." But I was desperate. At that point, if you had told me to go in the corner for two hours a day and stand on my head, I would have done it to feel better. I couldn't live like that for much longer. It was wearing on every single part of me. So I started getting chiropractic care.

I was so thankful when my back started feeling better. I could move and be without pain. What a relief! Then one day it hit me. When had my last headache been? I looked back and realized it was seven days before, right before I started treatment. *No way—pure coincidence.*

Then ten days went by. I was in a panic. Like so many of you, I had been told by one of my esteemed doctors that it was all in my head (don't you just love that?). Still, even though I knew it wasn't, I started to panic, thinking *what if I made this all up?* I made myself a deal: if I made it two weeks with no headache, I was going to say something. Besides, one way or the other, I didn't want to jinx it. Sure enough, two weeks came with no headaches. I finally decided to say something to the chiropractor. I remember the conversation like it was yesterday. He put a "normal" X-ray on the board and showed me how it was supposed to look. How from the side there was supposed to be this C-shaped kind of curve. Then he put mine up there.

"What do you think, Rob?" he asked me. "It's backwards; my C goes in the wrong direction," I replied, pretty sure that it was a trick question. He was happy to tell me how right I was and that in his opinion it was the cause of all my headaches. I was flabbergasted. I told him that it was impossible, that I had had dozens of X-rays and scans and no one had said anything about that to me. He went on to explain that it was there all along, even if nobody credited it for causing my problem. It was putting pressure on my nerves and causing the symptoms of my headaches. Remember, I was fourteen years old. I didn't know what to think. All I knew was that I didn't have a headache for the longest stretch in four years and, while I wasn't a great radiologist at that point in my life, I knew that my X-ray didn't look like that normal one.

That was over twenty years ago and I haven't had a headache since. It made a tremendous difference in my life, but not in the way you would think. Sure, it was nice to feel better, but I was more interested in what I had just discovered. For the first time in dealing with health care, I found something where I could say, "Yeah, that makes sense." I watched people go to this doctor and leave his office happier and healthier than when they went in. I took every pamphlet he had. I read it all. I asked a ton of questions. Finally the doctor (who I am assuming did this out of self-preservation so I would quit badgering him) offered to take me to a seminar on natural healing. I accepted not knowing what to expect.

My father and I went to this giant hall and watched all these different doctors go up on stage and talk. We were the only non-doctors there. All I could think as one after another got up there and spoke was, "This all makes sense." It was logical. I could wrap my mind around it. Could it really be this simple, this straightforward cause-and-effect concept? When I got in the car with my father after it was over, I told him, "Dad, this is what I'm going to do with my life." I never looked back and my journey started that night.

I tore through chiropractic school just in love with the concept that in natural medicine the body could heal itself. Soon I graduated and immediately opened up my own practice. I was on purpose and fulfilling my mission. I was helping people. I wanted to help every single last one of them, no matter how complicated the problem was. Then one day something hit me in the face like a ton of bricks.

If the body could and should heal itself, then why, in really complicated cases, didn't it? We would adjust our patients and maybe they would feel better, but the diabetics were still diabetics. The autoimmune patients still had autoimmune diseases. The really complicated chronic pain cases may have gotten temporary relief at best, but never resolved totally. Worse than all that, what drove me crazy was that there were no doctors out there helping these people. It was at that point I decided I was going to dedicate myself all over again to learning as much as I could about helping chronic conditions. One day I walked into the same advanced technique seminar as Dr. Katinka. We became friends and found out that we had the same purpose and were on a quest to help the most difficult cases. We spent the next four years traveling from seminar to seminar, learning and putting together all the pieces of the puzzle that we needed together. The rest, as they say, is history. Now, it is time for us to bring this work to you.

My clinic deals with the worst of the worst. We have patients travel to us from around the United States for care. I've won awards and been featured in magazines and newspapers. I even had a top government official from health and human services in Washington, DC, fly out to the grand opening of my newest clinic in Henderson, NV, just outside of Las Vegas. But at the end of the day none of that stuff matters. With what we know now, science is evolving to the point where the latest treatments are catching up to the latest research. These days, there are real solutions to these problems. What matters now is that when I sit down with my patients I can truthfully say to them, "You don't have to be sick anymore if you don't want to. Not on my watch."

RUNNING OUT OF FUEL

The war for your quality of life begins with the battle for your cells.

Let us look at what occurs on the cellular level that sets the stage for fibromyalgia to occur. I know it can get a bit scientific and complicated, but the basics of this information are absolutely vital when it comes down to who gets well and who doesn't. By the end of this chapter we will connect some dots and give you a practical step-by-step action guide incorporating all the material we have covered in this book. If you don't correct the faulty cellular processes, you will never be able to achieve the healing you are hoping for.

You probably remember way back in grade school science class when you learned about the cell. Every cell has its functions and every part plays a role. The nucleus of the cell acts as the brain, guiding the cell through what it needs to do. The mitochondria of the cell act as the power generator, driving the ability of the cell to create energy. The cell membrane is the outside covering of the cell that allows passage of materials in and out of the cell. Some of the most exciting breakthroughs have come in learning about the different roles of the cells, how they break down, and how they cause complex disease.

Fibromylagia is one of the main diseases discussed in all this new research.

I think it is clear by now that for fibromyalgia there usually isn't a single cause, but many factors combining. However, if you absolutely forced me to choose one reason why a human body would break down and become sick, my answer would be simple: the body simply could not create enough energy. With that in mind, while all the previous attention on the cellular function was looking at the nucleus, we have found that the answers to more of these problems lie in energy production in the mitochondria and the cellular membrane. In fact, if you remove the nucleus of a cell, the cell will live for another three months! But what happens if you remove the cell membrane? The cell dies instantly, putting up no fight. The diseases caused by these cell malfunctions have been classified as mitochondrial diseases, formerly known as "no cause, no cure."

We live and die at the cellular level. When our cells completely run out of energy, the body dies. When the cells run short of energy, the body becomes sick. The production of energy depends on the mitochondria to create adenosine triphosphate (ATP). Just as gasoline is the fuel that makes your car run, ATP is the fuel that your cell uses for every single process, from repair of DNA, to bringing nutrients into the cell and kicking toxins and metabolic wastes out. It's literally the currency that your body uses to conduct its business. Therefore, when the mitochondria become damaged, it is like a nuclear reactor meltdown that causes your body to not be able to create enough energy to heal; it will begin getting sick and continue down that path with no recourse. We spent a lot of time in an earlier chapter talking about the vitalistic approach to health. If the body was designed to heal itself, then why doesn't it? Simple. It ran out of the energy to do so.

What causes the mitochondria to become damaged and stop producing enough ATP for healing energy? Age? Sure, it is true that as we get older, the body tends to have fewer mitochondria available.

However, make no mistake, it really has nothing to do with age. Age is not a disease. All age really means in the health care equation is that the longer you have been around, the more chance you have to mess something up in your body and accumulate the bad things that will kill you. I've consulted thirty-year-olds who tell me they don't feel well because "they are getting older." Rest assured, age is not the key player here, no matter which doctor told you it was. The main reason mitochondria become damaged is that they are exposed to toxic chemicals that destroy their ability to function.

Most people would agree that we live in a toxic world. The environment around us exposes us to chemicals in the air we breathe, the water we drink and bathe in, and the food we eat. Interestingly enough, in my daily conversations with patients, while they will agree with the former statement, they often seem to be surprised when I suggest that those very same chemicals will accumulate in their bodies and cause them to become sick. Make no mistake about it, this chemical exposure is going to become the epidemic of our time.

Obviously we are fighting an external problem here. If somehow we could protect ourselves from chemicals in the outside world we would be safe, right? Well, this is where things get a little tricky. It turns out our health is being threatened from the *inside* too.

THE ROLE OF FREE RADICALS

Welcome to the world of free radicals, those nasty little unstable molecules in your body that, like termites in your house, will destroy it from the inside out. While outside chemicals can cause free radical damage, here lies the twist. When the mitochondria create ATP, they create *naturally* occurring free radicals as a by-product. Never fear, however, as the body in all its wisdom has a mechanism to deal with these molecules. How? The body uses antioxidants to neutralize the free radicals. So all is well, right? Unfortunately, due to the amount of chemicals we are exposed to from the environment and the fact that most people don't get enough nutrients from their diet, the body does not have enough antioxidants left over to neutralize both the free radicals created inside the cell naturally and the chemicals we are exposed to from the environment we live in. To further the problem, producing the major anti-oxidant that the body uses to fight this process (called glutathione) is incredibly energy-taxing. It takes four ATP just to create one glutathione. In a situation where energy is lacking to begin with, this is very energetically expensive.

As a result, the mitochondria are choking on the buildup of all these free radicals inside the cell. It can no longer produce enough ATP to provide the cell with all the energy that it needs to do its housekeeping. When the cell can't get the free radicals out and energy production is compromised, we refer to this process as inflammation. You are probably familiar with this word more than most, seeing that you walk around feeling like you are inflamed. Hearing that you most probably *are* inflamed should therefore come as no surprise.

However, when most people think of inflammation they think of something like a sprained ankle that gets red, swollen, and hot to the touch. That is describing extracellular inflammation, which happens outside the cells. As a fibromyalgia sufferer, your culprit is intracellular inflammation, meaning that every single cell in your body is inflamed. If you remember nothing else from this chapter, walk away thinking about the importance of controlling cellular inflammation in order to get better.[70]

OONO: THE SUPERVILLAIN INSIDE YOUR BODY

Inflammation is not always a bad thing. If you get a bacterial or viral infection, a physical trauma, or even severe psychological stress, your body will use a localized inflammation process starting with nitric oxide (NO). This is a really healthy response, and you might have heard that there is a medical treatment following the same idea where they give a heart attack victim "nitro" in order for them to survive. While it is very important in cardiovascular function, your immune system also uses NO to fight bacteria and viral infections.

However, if your body is not equipped with enough antioxidants that can get inside the cell and stop NO in its tracks, it combines with another free radical called super oxide and behold, one of the most toxic free radicals inside your body is born: peroxynitrite or OONO. Want more bad news? OONO has twenty-two different ways to create more NO, which in turn creates even more OONO. Can you see the vicious cycle that takes place? Antioxidants are like the bouncers who step in and break up the out-of-control bar fight. Without them, chaos ensues.[71,72,73]

WHEN CELLS MEMBRANES BECOME RESISTANT

You may rightfully wonder at this point whether simply supplementing with antioxidants would solve the issue. I wish it were that simple. However, there is another problem we haven't talked about yet. All that intracellular inflammation begins to lead to something called cell membrane resistance. This means that the cell membrane becomes unable to let waste products out of the cell, or nutrients into the cell—that includes antioxidants. Therefore, even if you take antioxidants, they most likely will not make their way *into* the cells, where they are really needed.

So this raises the question: what other nutrients cannot get into the cell if the cell membrane is inflamed and walled off? For type II diabetics, we call this insulin resistance. Insulin is not putting the glucose from the blood sugar into the cell to provide the fuel to make ATP. Insulin and leptin are the two primary hormones that end up unable to enter the cell through an inflamed membrane. Leptin may be a hormone that you are not familiar with, but you need to be.

Leptin is the hormone that tells the body to stop eating when it is full, as well as triggering the burning of fat for fuel. High levels of leptin in the blood indicate that it is unable to enter the brain cells of the hypothalamus and trigger appetite suppression and fat burning. Therefore, leptin resistance causes weight gain and the inability to burn fat. Insulin resistance causes food to be stored as fat, and leptin regulates the body's ability to burn fat. Hence the very same toxins that inflame the cell membranes coupled with the body's own hormones become "obesogens" and are the reason that so many people gain weight or struggle to lose weight.

METHYLATION

Hang on, because this may get technical. I will try to keep it simple. Methylation is a chemical reaction that occurs in every cell and tissue in the body. It is the process of adding a methyl group, consisting of one carbon and three hydrogen atoms, to another molecule. It plays a major role in many different functions, but for fibromyalgia it is important because of its interactions with proteins and neurotransmitters—the major reasons why your pain levels are so high and why you may suffer from depression.

Methylation of proteins helps the body detoxify. It will take a toxic amino acid called homocysteine (which is known to cause cardiovascular disease) and convert it into a beneficial amino acid called methionine. When methionine hooks up with ATP and magnesium, it forms SAM, which controls over four hundred chemical reactions in the body. You may have tried a supplement called SAM-E to help with sleep and mood regulation. Neurotransmitters are basically just amino acids with a methyl group attached to them. They are the chemicals that control our moods and how we feel and react. SAM-E is a precursor to seratonin, known as the "feel-good" hormone, which is almost always seen in reduced levels in fibromyalgia patients.

If a person is unable to methylate and there is a shortage of methyl groups, it will cause the "chemical imbalance" of depression. This sets off a cascade that will cause the adrenal glands to stay depleted and keep the hormones out of balance. It will cause the blood vessels to constrict, decreasing the flow of oxygen to the muscles and at the same time increasing the blood flow to the head. This not only explains the pressurized feeling in the head and headaches, but also the muscle pain.

Have you ever started an exercise program and felt soreness in your muscles? In fibro, this can even be more pronounced because of the issue of depleted methylation. The waste product of muscle performance is called lactic acid. As always, nature has a great plan to process lactic acid. If lactic acid production is normal, then when supplied with the right nutrients, ATP and oxygen, the body will begin to produce even more ATP. However, if there is a depletion of methyl groups to donate, it causes a shortage of oxygen in the muscles, causing them to get overwhelmed with lactic acid. The soreness will last for a much longer time until the liver and kidneys can remove the waste. This is why many doctors will recommend exercise to fibromyalgia patients, but without checking to see if they can methylate properly, it is a bad idea, and why so many fibromyalgia patients have increased pain for days after working out.

THE CHICKEN OR THE EGG?

We spent a lot of time and effort in previous chapters explaining how fibromyalgia is, at its basis, a neurological condition. So what comes first, the neurological problem or the cellular problem? While the answer is dependent on the injury that started it all, they are intimately related. When the nitric oxide cycle is out of control, it stimulates receptors called N-methyl-D-aspartate (or NMDA) that have an excitatory response on the autonomic nervous system. The ability of the mitochondria to even begin to produce ATP is completely driven by the autonomic nervous system. An inability to methylate causes an instability of the autonomic nervous system and never allows the system to reset itself. As you can see, regardless of how it happened, at the end of the day, in order to get better, you have to deal with it all these factors *together*.

CHAPTER 13

THE BRICK ROAD BACK TO HEALTH: A STEP BY STEP GUIDE

(DR. KATINKA VAN DER MERWE AND DR. ROBERT V. DEMARTINO)

"But it is a long way to the Emerald City, and it will take you many days. The country here is pleasant, but you must pass through rough and dangerous places before you reach the end of your journey."

This worried Dorothy a little, but she knew that only the great Oz could help her get to Kansas again, so she bravely resolved not to turn back
                                    —L. Frank Baum, The Wizard of Oz

Your own resolution to succeed is more important than any other one thing.
                                    —Abraham Lincoln

*I have heard there are troubles of
more than one kind.
Some come from ahead and some
come from behind.
But I've bought a big bat. I'm all
ready, you see.
Now my troubles are going to have
troubles with me!*

—*Dr. Seuss*

Please remember that the steps discussed below are part of a very specific system or recipe. If you follow a chocolate chip cookie recipe, you can't decide to cherry-pick ingredients and expect to end up with the same cookies. Every treatment we chose was carefully selected from all around the world, and added with forethought after much research. We do not claim to cure fibromyalgia. We treat bodies, not symptoms, and systems, not individual organs. We have noticed that following the treatment plan below, a large number of our patients who suffer from fibromyalgia experience a dramatic improvement in their neurological symptoms.

In our clinics, we use a three-tiered approach to patient care: functional medicine, physical medicine, and neurological rehabilitation. In order to accomplish this, we use a combination of the Neurological Relief Center technique to balance and correct any autonomic nervous system imbalances, quantum neurology (a system developed by Dr. George Conzalez from Los Angeles, used to rehabilitate the nervous system), detoxification, heavy metal testing, biological medicine, and frequency-specific microcurrent, a new system of treatment using microamperage current. The resulting resonance effects of frequencies on tissues and conditions to create beneficial changes in symptoms and health are proven to be effective for inflammation in the case of fibromyalgia.[69]

While many of our patients travel to us for care from across the world, we understand that this isn't possible for everyone. That is why we will try to outline the steps necessary to take when healing the neurological and physical symptoms associated with fibromyalgia. We are very conscious that these steps are not simple, and this is not an easy do-it-yourself guide. We wish that were possible, but fibromyalgia is a complicated condition that requires complicated solutions.

While designing these steps was a daunting task, it was also an exciting one. There has never been a better time to suffer from fibromyalgia, if you have to suffer from it. The treatment options that we now have available to us allow us to effectively evaluate and change what caused the problem in the first place, giving us real hope and real results. If there is a silver lining in having fibromyalgia, it is that there are now options to get better that just didn't exist in the past.

With that being said, it is not all sunshine and rainbows. It takes tremendous hard work to get better. Unfortunately, there is no magic pill and there will never be one. Hopefully, after going through all the science in this book, it will become apparent why we say that there will never be a drug that "cures" fibromyalgia. In these types of complex disease processes, only a complex treatment program will bring about true healing. It takes time to heal. Trust us, we also wish there were a simple solution to fibromyalgia. As doctors, it would be so much easier to treat and get results, but that is just not the case. In our opinion, any book or supplement that promises a simple solution is misleading.

By now it should be apparent that it takes time for all of these problems to progress to the levels they are at now. It takes a millisecond to step off a curb wrong and break your ankle, but it takes six weeks to heal. It is not really fair, but there is no healing process that does not require time. The good news is, as you heal you should begin to feel better. However, it will not happen overnight.In addition to time, it takes effort. It is not the easiest thing in the world to change your diet. It makes dining out harder and sometimes you may feel like you are being deprived or punished. You may even feel worse before you start feeling better. But you need to do it in order to get better.

While it is possible, in many cases fibromyalgia cannot be corrected without some help. When we took on the task of writing this book, people kept asking us to make a "self-help" book. Unfortunately, in most cases (not all, people have recovered themselves) you will need help with getting well from medical providers who are in the know about fibro. So there will be a cost to getting well, and it may be significant. If you suffered from cancer or some other life-threatening condition, cost would usually quickly become a minor obstacle, as people will do whatever it takes.

Make no mistake about it: fibromyalgia is life-threatening too. It may not be fatal, but it can rob the quality of your life until there is not much left. Now, it is not our place to tell you how to spend your money or give you financial advice. We just want to be totally transparent here. The old cliché is that you cannot put a price tag on your health. Well, unfortunately, that is exactly what you are going to have to do.

In a final word on this, the major difference between the people who succeed in getting better and the people who don't comes down to a single word: consistency. Just as with anything in life, whether it is work or relationships, the people who are consistent in actions that will move them forward go in the direction that they want. Take a good look at where your life is and where you would like it to be. Hold that vision and decide right now if you will do whatever it takes to get it where you want it. Excuses and difficult circumstances will always be there. Consistently decide to let nothing throw you off your goal to get your life back.

We not only did a tremendous amount of research to bring you this book, but we also conferred with our patients and support groups that we work with to find out what you wanted in a fibromyalgia book and what you felt was lacking. The number one answer was this: after they finished reading the book, people were excited about the possibility of getting better but didn't know the steps to take to get there. Where do I start? What do I do? Where do I go from here?

This is what is called the Jacuzzi effect. When you are in the Jacuzzi you feel great, much like being excited about reading the info in this book. But when you get out, you feel about the same as when you got in. You feel cold. That good feeling evaporates with the water. That is not what we wanted for you. So we designed action steps and options for you to follow in order to facilitate your recovery. Let these steps guide you toward healing.

On our website, www.tamethefibrobeast.com, you will find all the tests and packages you will need to complete steps 2 and 3. You will also be able to book consultations with us, and find additional information. We wanted to be able to help people who are unable to travel to us due to money, obligations, distance or poor health. We also wanted you to empower yourself, and take back control from your doctors. Make sure to read this book in its entirety before embarking on these steps. Part of our commitment is to constantly update our website with the latest research, information, supplementation and techniques. It is much easier to update our website often rather than this book.

THE SYSTEM:
A STEP-BY-STEP GUIDE

Step One: Balance the Autonomic Nervous System If Necessary

As we were talking about when listing all of the different types of fibromyalgia, the initial step is to figure out what the major players are that are lcausing your problem. Get to a doctor who can physically evaluate the structures of your neck. This may even require some motion X-ray evaluations to determine if you are experiencing stenosis or structural damage (please refer to chapter 5). If you have these already, consult a doctor who knows something about correcting the problem. If you have problems in your cervical spine, we highly recommend that you consult with a doctor who is trained in detecting problems with and in balancing the autonomic nervous system gently and effectively.

This process will take time (in our clinics usually about ten to twelve weeks). This step is crucial, and if you don't have a doctor near you, it is worth traveling for. The good news is that if your fibromyalgia is caused by cervical trauma or an imbalance of the autonomic nervous system, you will frequently see changes in your neurological symptoms very fast while being treated with this technique. We recommend twice-a-month maintenance visits to our patients after they complete their care whenever possible. Go to www.nrc.md to find out if there is a doctor near you.

Please note that if there is no doctor near you trained in this technique, and you are unable to travel to one for care, that we recommend that you proceed to the next step, and test and treat at home with our guidance and support. Go to www.tamethefibrobeast.com for more information.

Step Two: Get Tested (All test kits available on www.tamethefibrobeast.com)

You need to get evaluated not only on the physical level, but also on the chemical and cellular level. While it is safe to say that most of these problems are typically occurring, it is also necessary to get baselines on your current status to make sure that you are getting the results that you want as you progress. That way, you can measure your progress. The tests that we typically recommend are the following:

- **Heavy metal screening test** (we recommend a urine test).

  ○ If positive, we recommend taking the following products under the supervision of a knowledgeable doctor as necessary: Metal Free by Body Health or ULTRA Liquid Zeolite™.

◦ It is best to "cycle" while detoxing from heavy metals, meaning you take the product every four hours for four days and then stop taking it for ten days (repeat as necessary and please consult your doctor.)

◦ We also recommend that you consult with a biologic dentist if you have had amalgam fillings, root canals, or other metal placed in your mouth. (Please refer to chapter 5.)

- **Lipid peroxidation testing** for measuring the level of cellular inflammation and cell membrane damage (if positive please go to www.tamethefibrobeast.com to find out more about our cellular inflammation kit.)

- **Nitric oxide testing.** Determines the level of nitric oxide involvement in mitochondrial dysfunction (if positive, please go to www.tamethefibrobeast.com to order the NO/ONOO kit.)

- **Dysbiosis test** to determine if there is leaky gut syndrome. (If positive, please go to www.tamethefibrobeast.com to order the gut rebuild kit.)

- **pH testing** to determine the acid/alkaline ratios in the body (please alkalize your diet and consider taking a good quality barley green supplement if acidic.)

- **Visual Contrast testing** to evaluate the eyes' ability to see contrast. Specific biotoxins may trigger a cascade of effects in the body, causing autoimmune conditions and inflammation. It may prevent the neurologic symptoms of fibromyalgia from healing. If a person has a biotoxic illness (mold exposure, heavy bacterial or viral infection) it will compromise their ability to see contrast. The test is very accurate and noninvasive for getting a measurement in that capacity. The link for this test is on our website. (If positive, please go to www.tamethefibrobeast.com to order the biotoxin kit.)

- **Thyroid and adrenal testing** (Please refer to chapter 8 to see exactly which tests to order.) If you order these tests through your doctor, your insurance may cover a portion of the test, or the entire test, depending on your insurance coverage. However, you may also order this test from www.privatemdlabs.com (order the thyroid deluxe package), although you will have to pay out of pocket for this test.

A brief word about these tests: Many of these tests require no blood work. Some can be done by blood work, but be wary of the results that they show. For example, if your doctor did a blood test for heavy metal poisoning, unless you had a recent major exposure, it would come up negative. So many times people bring us "normal" blood work even though they are sick. Their doctors either missed certain tests or their specific problems are not accurately diagnosed by blood. We prefer urine (or stool, but urine is easier) to evaluate most problems. For metal, lipid peroxidation, and leaky gut they are the best diagnostic tools we have.

As I am sure you have found in the past, it is difficult to find a doctor who orders this type of testing. Many don't even know that it exists. You may end up going to more than one doctor's office to get different tests. So here is what we decided to do to help you:

You can order home versions of these tests on our website www.tamethefibrobeast.com, and book a consultation with

one of our doctors. After taking the test, and consulting with one of our doctors about your individual test results, you will have the opportunity to sign up for our six month coaching program designed for your individual needs. This program will allow you to have access to the nutritional plans, supplements, fibromyalgia specific diet and programs that we use for our patients in our clinics in order to solve issues like cellular inflammation, leaky gut, mitochondrial dysfunction, methylation, and the like.

Please do not misunderstand what we are trying to do here. You are certainly welcome to go out there and try to put this all together on your own. It can be done. We will encourage you to find a team of professionals who are all on the same page and will help in your journey of healing, using the guidelines set forth in this book. We listened to all your feedback up to now and are trying to make a complicated issue as simple as possible. We designed it so you would have another option to get additional help. Nothing more, nothing less.

Step Three (moving into maintenance): Take the Supplements Suggested In This Book

If the tests above are positive and you have to choose between purchasing the repair kits and the supplements mentioned in this book, we suggest that you purchase the kits until your test(s) are negative and then move on to taking the supplements. If the cellular membranes are faulty, it is very difficult to get good nutrition inside the cell. Therefor, we suggest the above tests and kits (if positive) before moving into supplementation.

Step Four: Change Your Diet (80 percent of the rest of your life)

Please refer to chapter 11. Do not put off the changes you can make today until tomorrow. Remember, in a nutshell, your basic goals with your diet should be to add to your health. You are going to try to alkalize your pH, eat lots of fresh fruits and vegetables, eat less animal protein (grass or pasture fed if possible), cut down on carbs (especially unhealthy ones) and include good healthy fats. Also, you are going to be a good patient and avoid the things on the no-no list, as described in chapter 11. Eating healthfully should become a lifestyle for you. Do *not* call it a diet. It is not a temporary change.

Remember, getting better is a journey, not a race. You have to accept that along this journey, you may have peaks as well as valleys. I always remind my patients that if you could picture healing as a line on a graph, it would not be a straight line that is steadily climbing, but rather a line with "waves" in it. What you must look for and celebrate are the times that you feel better increasing, both in number and duration, and the bad days decreasing in the same manner. If it were easy, everybody would get better.

It is not easy, cheap, or simple, but it is possible. It is the way back to Kansas.

CHAPTER 14

DON'T. YOU. EVER. GIVE. UP.

To disprove the theory that all crows are black,
you only need to find one white crow.
　　　　　　—Professor William James, Harvard

Whether you think you can, or you
think you can't—you're right.
　　　　　　　　　　　—Henry Ford

If fifty million people say a foolish
thing, it is still a foolish thing.
　　　　　　　　　　—Anatole France

I have a very specific way of interviewing every new patient who walks through my clinic doors. When a patient "hires" me, they hand me their trust, and because of it, I feel a tremendous amount of responsibility. Healing is a journey, and they hire me to be their guide. With every patient, we first establish a goal, a reason for fighting. If you undertake a journey, you need a destination. Most suffering from fibromyalgia have forgotten what it feels like to be healthy. The patient needs something to "anchor" them back in the world of the healthy—a reason, a goal, or a powerful motivation.

Usually, the most important question I ask a new patient on their first day of treatment is this: "What do you miss the most about being healthy? What is it that you wish you could do and can't do anymore because of fibromyalgia?" That answer means so much to me as a doctor. You see, I am very goal-oriented, and I believe that both my patient and I need a reason to fight their way back to health. Fighting that fight is not easy, and it is not for everyone. Taming the beast that is fibromyalgia takes courage, grit, tenacity, and a warrior spirit. Like we said earlier, it is not a sprint, but a marathon.

It is *so* worth trying, however. What do you miss the most about being healthy? Picking up your grandchild? Being a good mom? Going to a football game with your family? Waking up without pain? Going back to work? It is possible to forget how good life can be without daily pain, but you mustn't allow yourself to do so. You have to fight. I am of the opinion that the number one predictor that a patient will get better is their attitude.

I wish I could count the times that I have been hotly reprimanded and debated at lectures, online, or in my practice, by people suffering from fibromyalgia. Basically, they all say the same thing: "But there is no cure for fibromyalgia! Who are you to say it could get better? Are you smarter than all these experts and researchers and doctors?" To this, I like to quote my father, who often uses a quote by a professor from Harvard named William Jones: "To disprove the theory that all crows are black, you only need to find one white crow." I have seen people suffering from fibromyalgia find their way back to health. I have seen a white crow.

This is an extremely subjective and sensitive topic. When the word "cure" is used, that brings to mind visions of a miracle pill, injection, or surgery studied and proven by perhaps a promising double-blind study and excitedly announced by the media. Please believe me when I tell you that it won't happen that way. The failure in finding such a "cure" lies in the theory of what fibromyalgia is, or what it is caused by. It is a complex problem, not a puzzle with a single solution. It is not a condition that can be healed by a miracle chemical; it is a body where a whole bunch of things went wrong.

Fibromyalgia must be approached by a method where every system involved is checked and rebuilt, if necessary, in a systematic way. I've personally known numerous patients and acquaintances who consider themselves healed from fibromyalgia. I have heard people tell their stories about finding their own recoveries in their own ways on the Internet. I have seen it with my own eyes, and I have seen these patients stay better. If even one patient can do it, why can't you?

Of course, I understand that when the medical community tells the world that patients can't recover from fibromyalgia, it becomes easy to believe that as gospel truth. I also understand that many of you have been taken advantage of by ruthless vultures or misguided people. Some may think they can help, or want to help, but in the end change nothing except emptying your pockets. I would imagine that after a while, that can make you bitter.

We do not claim to have found a cure for fibromyalgia. What we do know is that we have found a way to treat the *neurological symptoms* associated with fibromyalgia successfully. It is our way, but may not be the only way. The number one thing you need to do when you examine any new treatment is to speak to other patients who have undergone that treatment. Did it work for them? How long did it work for? You must be your own best advocate. As the late president Ronald Reagan used to say, "Trust, but verify." Do not enter treatments or take supplements or medications blindly. Always do your due diligence.

The number one thing all successful patients have in common is hope. Hope allows patients to still try, and to do what they have to do in order to get better. It has been said that a sign of insanity is doing the same thing over and over, expecting a different outcome. If you are sick today, it is clear that what you have been doing up to now is not working and that it is time to approach your condition differently. Patients who assume responsibility for their own health care challenges, then do their own research and are willing to do what it takes, *can* make dramatic improvements. If you suffer a great deal, which is true for most people with fibromyalgia, even long-term decrease of your pain by 30 percent can feel like a massive relief. Never, ever give up.

NOREEN'S STORY

My name is Noreen Williams and this is my fibromyalgia story. My journey with fibro began over thirty years ago with an accident resulting in my first of seven head injuries. Over the years my symptoms of intense pain, headaches, depression, female problems, stomach issues, and intense fatigue and other ailments became more "normal" than feeling good. I was adopted into a large family with a very strict work ethic. I learned early that hard work was rewarding in many ways, including financially, and started working for neighbors at age nine so I could have my own money. I also learned to ignore pain and just keep going, to be tough and never let others know if there was something wrong.

I also learned to be a major caregiver at a very early age, so I was even more aware of putting others' needs ahead of my own! I worked my way through nursing school and began a very rewarding career as an RN. I made it twenty years and then my body suddenly went on strike; I could not get out of bed due to the severity of all the fibro symptoms. Six months prior to this, I had my seventh head injury when a truck rear-ended me at a stoplight. After this accident, I just could not seem to manage my symptoms any longer. Everything spiraled out of control. Before this, I had been able to somehow still work while juggling pain, depression, IBS symptoms, eye problems, balance issues, major memory problems, and brain fog.

Over the years I had tried nutritional and vitamin supplements and many new "promises of a cure" for fibro or pain. I had been to three different lifestyle-change programs that had me away from home three to four weeks at a time. I tried exercise, diets, water and light therapies, yoga/relaxation, and massage. You name it.

Then there were the drugs, experimental therapies, psych consults, doctor visits, and being told to just "suck it up." So many meds I didn't want to take and then the side effects too numerous to mention! So here I am in 2004 earning a great salary, loving my job, family, and friends, busy with life—and then I can't function because my body has shut down. I finally got disability after fighting for three years and losing everything in the process.

Over time I just got worse. I was in so much pain, even on numerous meds, that I just stayed in bed and cried. Light hurt my head, noise hurt me all over, movement hurt, and then there were all the other symptoms like diarrhea, nausea, throwing up, headaches, itchy skin, frequent urination, depression, weight loss, weakness, brain fog, inability to make decisions, and other symptoms. My family and friends knew that I was not doing well and were trying everything they knew to help me.

Several friends had heard of and gone to see Dr. Katinka. They would call and tell me about her and the great results she was having with fibro patients. I just thought, "I am so tired. I give up. Nothing has worked and I just don't have it in me to ever go check it out." I really felt that I was going to die in the next several months and had made final arrangements and told my family good-bye. That's how sick I was.

My husband finally said, "I need you to make the appointment so I can take you. If it doesn't work, I won't ask you to try anything else and I will let you go." I made the appointment. I could hardly talk on the phone at this time, so it took some time to do this, but we went to the appointment. I was so nervous and didn't know what to expect.

Dr. Katinka examined me and told me that first, we had to establish whether my neck problems had anything to do with my pain. She said that if they were connected, I might have significant (although not permanent, at first) relief from my pain. She was right. After the first treatment I felt absolutely incredible. After the treatment I went from pain levels higher than a ten to barely a twinge. I had two hours of feeling energetic and just the twinge of discomfort. I was euphoric, to say the least. Wow! That's when I knew I would get better. How much better, I had no idea. But I knew I would get better! I followed her treatment plan to a T.

Dr. Katinka gave me my life back. Not my previous life, but a life where I function and enjoy my family, friends, church, and community. I have learned that stress of any kind has a huge impact on fibro. My previous Type A work style, take-charge attitude, and lack of balance in my life contributed in a huge way to my decline. Life is stressful but can be managed if we are aware of the stressors and have coping mechanisms in place. I am so grateful that my family and friends made it possible for Dr. Katinka to treat me and to make me able to be part of life again! It has been two and a half years since I finished my treatment program. We are now raising a beautiful one-and-a-half-year-old granddaughter who has epilepsy. That would never have been possible if not for Dr. Katinka.

Please know there is hope! Give Dr. Katinka a chance; you have nothing to lose except your pain, and the opportunity to gain your life back. Good luck to you!

CHOOSE YOUR SUPPORT WISELY

While a great support group can be a wonderful thing, you must be very picky when choosing your support groups and those people in your inner circle. While you can't choose your family, you can choose your friends, support system, and doctors. If you find yourself encouraged and hopeful after interacting with someone, that is a good sign. A support group can be a very useful tool, if you find the right one. While it is great to commiserate about your pain and daily struggles with those who understand, you must also surround yourself with people who are open-minded and willing to support you in your journey to get well. If a group is negative or confrontational in any way, please steer clear.

WHAT YOU FOCUS ON EXPANDS

Let's pretend that you are healthy and one day, while sitting around, you get the crazy idea to complete a marathon. Say you are not a runner and frankly a bit of a couch potato. What would you guess is the best way to start? I'd say, turn to Google. That is my first step these days. Do you Google "ten reasons that most people will never finish a marathon"? No! You go and look for tips. Advice. You follow other people who have finished marathons. Perhaps you get a coach—someone who has experience and comes highly recommended, since they have coached other people from the couch over the finish line. You get my drift. What you give time, energy, and focus to will grow in your life.

Please keep the goal of recovering alive in your heart and mind. It has been done by others. It could be done by you. Do not allow negative people around you if you can help it. Minimize the input of those you can't avoid. In other words, let their words enter one ear, and exit the other.

POINTING THE BONE

This is an old practice among the Aborigine natives from Australia where a witch doctor (known as a Kurdaitcha) points a bone at a tribe member as punishment for some crime. Everyone in the village knows that this means certain death. The belief is so strong that within a few days, the hapless victim grows listless and refuses water and food, quickly dying, with no apparent cause besides the fatal pointing of that bone. Now, imagine if your doctor is not a witch doctor but a doctor wearing a white coat, working at one of the most prestigious hospitals in the United States, and he just told you that fibromyalgia has no cure...you get my drift.

The following is so important that I am repeating it. Your doctor needs to be well-informed, willing to listen, and keeping an open mind. Like we said earlier in this book, if your doctor has the nerve or audacity in this day and age, with all the research available to them, to tell you that the fibromyalgia you suffer from is all in your head, for heaven's sake, fire them. There is no excuse for that. It is not your job to convince them that you are not lying, looking for attention, or unwell psychologically.

> *"It matters not how strait the gate,*
> *How charged with punishments the scroll,*
> *I am the master of my fate:*
> *I am the captain of my soul."*
> — *William Ernest Henley*

PARTING WORDS OF WISDOM

1) **Plug in:** Find a way you can recharge every day. It is so easy to become isolated when you struggle alone just to get by. I

highly suggest meditation (not a "new age" practice, but a well-researched, well-established way to quiet your mind and recharge). I like the book *Getting In the Gap* by Dr. Wayne W. Dyer as a way to get started. If you believe in prayer, pray every day. If your spiritual life is important, practice it. Listen to music you love. Keep fresh flowers next to your bed. Do whatever you need to do to stay positive. Think of yourself as a rechargeable electric device. You need to stay energized, and that energy needs to come from somewhere.

2) **Ruthlessly cut out negative people who do not support your fight for recovery:** Unless, of course, they are family, and even then you should minimize your contact with them as much as possible. In their case, put on your invisible "Teflon" coat, so all their verbal arrows just bounce off of you. If you have toxic friends, acquaintances, or support groups, cut them loose. You cannot afford negativity in your life.

3) **Stop apologizing for being sick:** It's not your fault.

4) **Study those who got well:** If you run into other fibromyalgia sufferers in your support groups or other circles who say that they have recovered to some degree, ask them questions. Do not automatically assume that they are full of it.

5) **Become your own advocate:** Your health is your responsibility. It is absolutely irresponsible to hand over your most precious possessions (your body and your health) to your doctor, blindly trusting them. You should research every treatment, every medication, and every supplement suggested to you. Do not just Google the official websites either, but look up, for example, "Drug X side effects." That way, you will connect with ten thousand actual people who took or are taking drug X, discussing their own experiences with it.

6) **Become a researcher:** Stay on top of your condition. Do not expect your doctor to do this for you. With the Internet at your fingertips, this is not as hard as it used to be. Try using Google Scholar when looking for the latest research. For example, just type in "Irritable Bowel Syndrome Fibromyalgia." The research is always dated. Not all articles are free, but many are.

7) **You have the right to be supported:** Consider your condition to be a serious one. Sometimes, when so many doubt you, you may start doubting yourself. While it is good to stay positive, please do not feel the need to pretend that you feel good all the time. When you stuff all that pain down where others can't see it, you only do more damage. If people around you offer their support, accept it. Try to find others in the same boat to whom you can vent every now and then.

8) **Keep your mind in a healing consciousness:** My opinion here might not be popular, but I stand firmly by it. If you decide that you will never get better and that fibromyalgia will be your lifelong companion, the chances are that you are right. You have to keep on fighting, keep an open mind, keep researching, and keep your eyes and ears open for new developments.

9) **Approach your body as a unit, not a bunch of parts:** Start understanding how one part connects with another part. Develop a basic philosophy and appreciation for how the body works and how intelligent it is. Rebuild and heal it as a unit.

10) **Be kind to your body:** To the extent that you can, support your body with good food, good water, sunshine, and love.

11) **Try not to isolate yourself from the world:** When you need a hug, ask for one. When you are having a bad day, share that.

Try to interact with your friends and loved ones as much as you can, even if it means that you are just watching a movie with them on the couch in your PJs. Even getting some of you is still better for them than none of you at all.

12) **Give all disciplines of health care an equal shot:** I have run into this often. People often seem disappointed that I am not a medical doctor. "Oh. You're a chiropractor." Don't be a health care snob! Remember that long before the allopathic profession came around to the idea that fibromyalgia is a real condition, many alternative disciplines worked with fibromyalgia and considered it to be a real thing. No matter what the letters behind their name says, it is my opinion that doctors and other professionals learn what *really* matters after they graduate, through experience and postgraduate studies. A doctor is only as valuable as their knowledge. Your guide to health may not be a medical doctor, or even a doctor. Research their results, and make sure that they are knowledgeable and good at what they do.

While you and I may never meet, I want you to know that I truly care about you. People like you, suffering daily and living in agony, are what drives me and motivates me. I am sorry this condition happened to you, but I also know that there is a good chance that you may beat this thing. One of the best things that you may gain from this is that if you *do* get better, you will have a more intense appreciation and love for your health, and you will most likely never take it for granted again, the way healthy people do.

Remember, you are not alone. Millions of others have walked in your shoes. There *are* doctors who care about you, such as myself. Personally, I will never stop fighting for you, will never stop learning, and will never stop sharing what I learn with you. I have so much respect for what you have been through, and the fight that you have to fight in order to get better.

> *"To reach (our goal), we must sail sometimes with the wind and sometimes against it. But we must sail and not drift, not lie at anchor."*
> —*Oliver Wendell Holmes Sr., physician*
>
> *"Don't deny the diagnosis; try to defy the verdict."*
> —*Norman Cousins*

It is my most sincere wish for you that your journey back to health ultimately has a happy ending. I also wish you much happiness, joy, and many good pain-free days. After all, isn't life for the living?

Be strong, don't give up, and keep fighting like a warrior, for that is what you truly are. Do not let fibromyalgia define you; let fighting it define you.

THE END

REFERENCES

[1] R. Rogers, *Clinical Assessment of Malingering and Deception, 2nd ed.* (New York, NY: Guilford Press, 1997)

[2] Richard H. Gracely et al., *Functional magnetic resonance imaging evidence of augmented pain processing in fibromyalgia* (Article first published online May 8, 2002)

[3] M. Martínez-Lavín, *The Autonomic Nervous System and Fibromyalgia. The Clinical Neurobiology of Fibromyalgia and Myofascial Pain: Therapeutic Implications* (Binghamton, NY: The Haworth Press, 2002), 221-228

[4] J. Bruce Moseley et al., "A Controlled Trial of Arthroscopic Surgery for Osteoarthritis of the Knee," *Engl J Med* (2002)

[5] Vadim Gerasimov, *Information Processing in Human Body* (Based on final project for MIT Class MAS 862, 1998). Corrected and updated in 2000-2006

[6] Herbert A. Roberts, *The Principles and Art of Cure by Homœopathy,* p.156-162 (Suppression) 2002

[7] *Taber's Cyclopedic Medical Dictionary, 13th edition*

[8] Buskila et al., *Arthritis and Rheumatism* 40(3): 446-452, March 1997

[9] Seletz, "Whiplash Injuries," *JAMA* <u>Vol 168, No. 13</u> (1958)

[10] Mohamed B. Abou-Donia et al. *Splenda Alters Gut Microflora and Increases Intestinal P-Glycoprotein and Cytochrome P-450 in Male Rats* (Version of record first published: *Journal of Toxicology*, 18 Sep 2008)

[11] P. Roy-Byrne et al., "Post-traumatic stress disorder among patients with chronic pain and chronic fatigue," *Psychol Med* (2004)

[12] D. Buskila et al., *Increased rates of fibromyalgia following cervical spine injury. A controlled study of 161 cases of traumatic injury* (University of the Negev, Beer Sheva, Israel, 1997)

[13] Dan S. Heffez et al., *Can spinal cord compression cause the fibromyalgia syndrome?* (Chicago Institute of Neurosurgery and Neuroresearch, 1999)

[14] P. Matsuura et al., *Comparison of computerized tomography parameters of the cervical spine in normal control subjects and spinal cord-injured patients* (Regional Spinal Cord Injury Care System of Southern California, Rancho Los Amigos Medical Center, 1989)

[15] D.S. Evangelopoulous et al., "Computerized Tomographic Morphometric Analysis of the Cervical Spine," *The Open Orthopedics Journal*, 2012

[16] E. Uayama et al., *A Japanese family with FEOM1-linked congenital fibrosis of the extraocular muscles type 1 associated with spinal canal stenosis and refinement of the FEOM1 critical region* (Received 3 December 2002: Received in revised form 3 February 2003: Accepted 21 February 2003)

[17] T. Sakou et al., *Genetic study of ossification of the posterior longitudinal ligament in the cervical spine with human leukocyte antigen haplotype* (Department of Orthopedic Surgery, Faculty of Medicine, Kagoshima University, Japan, 1994)

[18] N. Nonopen-Hietala et al., *Sequence variations in the collagen IX and XI genes are associated with degenerative lumbar spinal stenosis*

[19] R. Ader, N. Cohen, and D. Felten, *Psychoneuroimmunology: interactions between the nervous system and the immune system* (1995)

[20] R. Klein, P.A. Berg, "A comparative study on antibodies to nucleoli and 5-hydroxytryptamine in patients with fibromyalgia syndrome and tryptophan-induced eosinophilia-myalgia," *Journal of Molecular Medicine* (1994)

[21] Daniel Hollander, "Intestinal permeability, leaky gut, and intestinal disorders," *Current Gastroenterology reports, Volume 1* (1999)

[22] Gail K. Adler, Valdis F. Manfredsdottir, and Katharine W. Creskoff, "Neuroendocrine abnormalities in fibromyalgia," *Current Pain and Headache Reports* (2002)

[23] K.P. May et al., *Sleep apnea in male patients with the fibromyalgia syndrome* (Department of Rheumatology, Fitzsimons Army Medical Center, Aurora, Colorado, 1993)

[24] Michael Maes, "Inflammatory and oxidative and nitrosative stress pathways underpinning chronic fatigue, somatization and psychosomatic symptoms," *Current Opinion in Psychiatry* (2008)

[25] M. Martinez-Lavin, *Biology and therapy of fibromyalgia. Stress, the stress response system, and fibromyalgia* (National Institute of Cardiology, Mexico City, 2007)

[26] M. Passatore and S. Roatta, *Influence of sympathetic nervous system on sensorimotor function: whiplash associated disorders (WAD) as a model.* (Department of Neuroscience, Physiology Division, University of Torino Medical School, 2006)

[27] D.J. Reis, D.A. Ruggiero, and S.F. Morrison, *The C1 area of the rostral ventrolateral medulla oblongata. A critical brainstem region for control of resting and reflex integration of arterial pressure* (New York: Division of Neurobiology, Cornell University Medical College, 1989)

[28] K.A. Adebove, D.G. Emerton, and T. Hughes, *Cervical sympathetic chain dysfunction after whiplash injury* (Accident & Emergency Department, North Tees Health NHS Trust, Stockton-on-Tees, UK)

[29] J.R. Taylor and L.T. Twomey, *Acute injuries to cervical joints. An autopsy study of neck sprain* (Department of Anatomy and Human Biology, University of Western Australia, Nedlands, 1993)

[30] M. Sasamoto, H.B. Chen, and S. Tsukahara, *Autonomic nerves containing substance P in the aqueous outflow channels and scleral spur of the guinea pig* (Tamaho, Japan: Department of Ophthalmology, Yamanashi Medical University, 1999)

[31] H. Llu, P. W. Mantyh, and A.I. Basbaum. *NMDA-receptor regulation of substance P release from primary afferent nociceptors* (San Francisco: Departments of Anatomy and Physiology, and W. M. Keck Foundation Center for Integrative Neuroscience, University of California San Francisco, 1997)

[32] Glenn Affleck et al., *Sequential daily relations of sleep, pain intensity, and attention to pain among women with fibromyalgia* (Farmington: Department of Community Medicine, University of Connecticut School of Medicine, C. 1996)

[33] R. C. Veith et al., *Sympathetic nervous system activity in major depression. Basal and desipramine-induced alterations in plasma norepinephrine kinetics* (Seattle: Geriatric Research, Education, and Clinical Center (GRECC), 1994)

[34] Monica E. Jarrett et al., *Anxiety and Depression Are Related to Autonomic Nervous System Function in Women with Irritable Bowel Syndrome* (2003)

[35] Martha Clare Morris et al., "Dietary Copper and High Saturated and Trans Fat Intakes Associated with Cognitive Decline," *JAMA* (2006)

[36] P. Autier and S. Gandini, "Vitamin D supplementation and total mortality: a meta-analysis of randomized controlled trials," *Arch Intern Med.* (2007)

[37] Y. Sato et al., *Menatetrenone and vitamin D2 with calcium supplements prevent nonvertebral fracture in elderly women with Alzheimer's disease* (2005)

[38] O.F. Sendur et al., *Serum antioxidants and nitric oxide levels in fibromyalgia: a controlled study,* (Department of Physical Medicine and Rehabilitation, Adnan Menderes University Medicine School Hospital, Turkey, 2009)

[39] M. Aviram et al., "Pomegranate juice consumption for 3 years by patients with carotid artery stenosis reduces common carotid intima-media thickness, blood pressure and LDL oxidation," *Clinical Nutrition* (2004)

[40] Patrick Chariot and Olivier Bignani, "Skeletal muscle disorders associated with selenium deficiency in humans," *Muscle & Nerve* (2003)

[41] L. Yan et al., *Reduced coenzyme Q10 supplementation decelerates senescence in SAMP1 mice* (Shinshu University Graduate School of Medicine, 2006)

[42] R. Lister, "An open pilot study to evaluate the potential benefits of coenzyme Q10 combined with Ginkgo biloba extract in fibromyalgia syndrome," *The Journal of International Medical Research* (2002)

[43] M. Cordero et al., "Coenzyme Q10 distribution in blood is altered in patients with Fibromyalgia," *Clinical Biochemistry* (2009)

[44] M. Rossini et al., *Double-blind, multicenter trial comparing acetyl l-carnitine with placebo in the treatment of fibromyalgia patients* (Rheumatology Unit, University of Verona, Rheumatology Unit, University of Pisa; Rheumatology Unit, University of Naples; Rheumatology Unit, Ospedale "La Colletta," Arenzano; Rheumatology Unit, University of Siena; Rheumatology Unit, University of Cagliari Italy, 2007)

[45] J. E. Teitelbaum, Clarence Johnson, and John St. Cyr, "The Use of D-Ribose in Chronic Fatigue Syndrome and Fibromyalgia: A Pilot Study," *The Journal of Alternative and Complementary Medicine* (November 2006)

[46] I.J. Russell et al., "Treatment of fibromyalgia syndrome with Super Malic: a randomized, double-blind, placebo-controlled, crossover pilot study," *The Journal of Rheumatology* (1995)

[47] T. Appelboom and C. Mélot, *Flexofytol, a Purified Curcumin Extract, in Fibromyalgia and Gout: A Retrospective Study* (Erasme University Hospital, Medical School, University of Brussels, Brussels, Belgium, 2013)

[48] O. Sendur et al., "The relationship between serum trace element levels and clinical parameters in patients with fibromyalgia," *Rheumatol International* 2008

[49] M De Ruyter, <u>Michael Maes</u>, and I. Mihaylova, "Lower serum zinc in Chronic Fatigue Syndrome (CFS): Relationships to immune dysfunctions and relevance for the oxidative stress status in CFS," *Journal of Affective Disorders* (2006)

[50] R.V. Damadian and D. Chu, "The Possible Role of Cranio-Cervical Trauma and Abnormal CSF Hydrodynamics in the Genesis of Multiple Sclerosis," *Physiol. Chem. Phys. & Med. NMR* (2011)

[51] G. Vighi et al., "Allergy and the gastrointestinal system," *Clin ExpImmunol* (2008)

[52] T. Buffington, "Comorbidity of interstitial cystitis with other unexplained clinical conditions," *The Journal of Urology* (2004)

[53] A. Monaco et al., "Dysregulation of the Autonomous Nervous System in Patients with Temporomandibular Disorders: A Pupillometric Study," *PLOS One Open Peer Reviewed Journal (2012)*

[54] M. Strittmatter et al., *Autonomic Nervous System and Neuroendocrine Changes in Patients with Idiopathic Trigeminal Neuralgia*(Department of Neurology, University of the Saarland, Germany, 1996)

[55] Y. Sterner et al., "Prospective study of trigeminal sensibility after whiplash trauma," *J Spinal Disord*(2001)

[56] A.G. Guggisberg, C.W. Hess, J. Mathis," The Significance of the Sympathetic Nervous System in the Pathophysiology of Periodic Leg Movements in Sleep," *SLEEP* (2007)

[57] A. Wachman and D.S. Bernstein, "Diet and osteoporosis," *The Lancet* (1968)

[58] J. Vormann et al., "Supplementation with alkaline minerals reduces symptoms in patients with chronic low back pain," *Trace Elem Med Biol.* (2001)

[59] R.M. Walker and H. M. Linkswiler, *Calcium retention in the adult human male as affected by protein intake* (Department of nutritional sciences, University of Wisconsin, 1972)

[60] C.A. Daley et al., "A review of fatty acid profiles and antioxidant content in grass-fed and grain-fed beef," *Nutritional Journal* (2010)

[61] M. Marchello, *Nutrient Composition of Grass- and Grain-Finished Bison (North Dakota State University, Fargo, ND.* Great Plains Research 2001)

[62] P.I.P. Ponte et al., "Influence of Pasture Intake on the Fatty Acid Composition, and Cholesterol, Tocopherols, and Tocotrienols Content in Meat from Free-Range Broilers," *Poultry Science* (2008)

[63] K.L. Weaver et al., "The content of favorable and unfavorable poly-unsaturated fatty acids found in commonly eaten fish," *J Am Diet Assoc.*(2008)

[64] Y. Taki et al., "Breakfast Staple Types Affect Brain Gray Matter Volume and Cognitive Function in Healthy Children," *PLOS One* (2010)

[65] K. Oh et al., "Carbohydrate Intake, Glycemic Index, Glycemic Load, and Dietary Fiber in Relation to Risk of Stroke in Women," *American Journal of Epidemiology* (2005)

[66] S. Liu et al., *Fruit and vegetable intake and risk of cardiovascular disease: the Women's Health Study* (American Society of Clinical Nutrition, 2000)

[67] J.W. Lampe, *Health effects of vegetables and fruit: assessing mechanisms of action in human experimental studies* (American Society of Clinical Nutrition, 1992)

[68] G. Block, B. Patterson, A. Subar, "Fruit, vegetables, and cancer prevention: A review of the epidemiological evidence," *Nutrition and Cancer* (1992)

[67] U. Ravnskov, "Dietary fat intake and risk of stroke: Allegations about dietary fat are unfounded," *British Medical Journal* (2003)

[68] J. Wang, D.G. Jackson, and G. Dahl," The food dye FD&C Blue No. 1 is a selective inhibitor of the ATP release channel Panx1," *JGP* (2013)

[69] C. R. McMakin, W. M. Gregory, and T. M. Phillips, "Cytokine changes with microcurrent treatment of fibromyalgia associated with cervical spine trauma," *Bodywork and Journal of Movement Therapies* (2004)

[70] M.D. Cordero et al., "Clinical Symptoms in Fibromyalgia Are Better Associated to Lipid Peroxidation Levels in Blood Mononuclear Cells Rather than in Plasma," *PLOS One*

[71] P.P. Beckman and L. Liaudet, *Nitric oxide and peroxynitrite in health and disease* (2007)

[72] Martin Pall, *Unexplained Illnesses: Disease Paradigm for Chronic Fatigue Syndrome, Multiple Chemical Sensitivity, Fibromyalgia, Post-Traumatic Stress Disorder, and Gulf War Syndrome*

[73] Robin Mayfield, *It used to be easier to get people well: Keeping up with Inflammation*